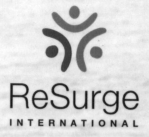

ReSurge
INTERNATIONAL

ReSurge International (formerly Interplast) is pleased to present to you this book about our work in 1998. Since then, our name has changed, but our mission to provide free reconstructive surgery to the world's poor continues.

the gift

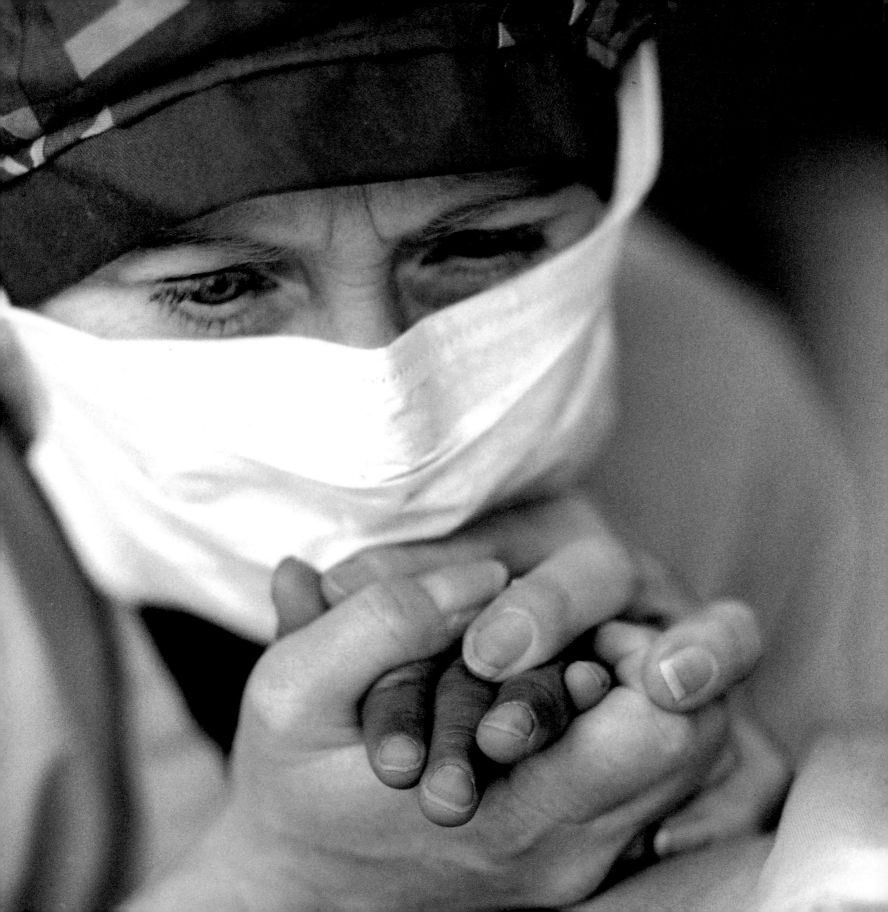

the gift

Phil Borges

Interplast, Inc.
Mountain View, California

Photographs copyright © 2000 by Phil Borges.
"For the Love of Children" copyright © 2000 by Diane Ackerman.
Compilation copyright © 2000 by Interplast, Inc.
All rights reserved.

The publisher gratefully acknowledges Diane Ackerman and Random House, Inc., for granting permission to adapt Ms. Ackerman's essay "For the Love of Children," originally published in *A Natural History of Love* (New York: Random House, 1994).

Library of Congress Catalog Card Number: 00-130137
ISBN: 0-9703998-0-4

For more information about supporting Interplast, contact:

Interplast, Inc.
300-B Pioneer Way
Mountain View, California 94041-1506
Tel: (650) 962-0123 • Fax: (650) 962-1619
IPNews@interplast.org • www.interplast.org
Interplast is a nonprofit, 501 (c) (3) organization.

Designed by Patrick David Barber
Produced by Marquand Books, Inc., Seattle
Printed and bound by CS Graphics Pte., Ltd., Singapore

contents

acknowledgments

AS INTERPLAST COMMEMORATES ITS 30TH ANNIversary, we extend our greatest thanks, admiration, and appreciation to the thousands of caring and dedicated volunteers, donors, and host-country colleagues who have made Interplast's work possible. The miracles documented in this book are but a few of the tens of thousands that your hands have created; on behalf of all those who have received your gift of new hope and new life, we dedicate this book to you.

We extend special thanks to Phil Borges for generously sharing his talents and his sensitive and extraordinary perspective to create this beautiful record of Interplast's work, and our heartfelt appreciation to Glen and Simone Anderson for making this book a reality.

We are deeply grateful to Diane Ackerman and Joan Baez for putting into words, as only they can, the emotions captured in these compelling photographs, and to Julee Geier, Ed Marquand, Patrick David Barber, Rachel Simpson, Mary Spillane, Marie Weiler, and Adam Woog for their commitment to and faith in this project, and their invaluable contributions, guidance, and support.

Finally, we wish to thank the following host colleagues and volunteers for their role in making this project possible, and our patients and their families for their extraordinary courage in allowing us to tell their stories:

Dr. Mario Cornejo Portillo

Dr. Tran Thanh Trai

Dr. Tran Van Do

Bradford Bohman, M.D.

Michael Champeau, M.D.

Paula Chandley, R.N.

Michael Cully, M.D.

Linh Doan, R.N.

Joan Don, M.D.

Gary Fudem, M.D.

Maureen Hanlon, R.N.

Jennifer Doan Hart

Sharon Henderson, R.N.

Terri Homer, M.D.

John Keiter, M.D.

Betty Kolbeck, R.N.

Kimberly Marble, M.D.

Lisa Mesner, R.N.

Julie Parker-Wing, R.N.

Barbara Platt, R.N.

Paul Rottler, M.D.

Jiwoong "John" Ryu, M.D.

Sunita Sastry, M.D.

Abby Smart, R.N.

Elaine Stasny, M.D.

Anthony Sudekum, M.D.

Alice Truscott, M.D.

Karen Yokoo, M.D.

Dawn Yost, R.N.

Stephen Yost

Alario, Leonardia, and
    José Luis

Nan and Hoi

Lucio and Isabel

Bay and Lien

Ester and Julia

Doithi and Lan

about Interplast

INTERPLAST, INC., IS A NONPROFIT ORGANIZATION that provides free reconstructive surgery for needy children in developing countries and medical education and training for host-country doctors and nurses.

Interplast schedules as many as forty surgical trips each year, sending teams of medical volunteers to sites in Bolivia, Brazil, Ecuador, Honduras, Laos, Myanmar, Nepal, Nicaragua, Peru, the Philippines, Tibet, and Vietnam. The teams provide nearly 3,000 free surgeries each year, treating children with such congenital birth defects as cleft lip and cleft palate, and children who have suffered severe burns or other crippling injuries. Interplast's volunteers work closely with local doctors and nurses to instruct them in advanced surgical techniques and related patient care, helping them improve their skills and become better able to provide these surgeries themselves. Interplast thereby leaves a lasting legacy, capable of touching the lives of thousands of children for generations to come.

Founded in 1969 by Dr. Donald R. Laub, then Chief of Reconstructive and Plastic Surgery at Stanford University Medical Center in Palo Alto, California, Interplast was the first organization of its kind. Through the efforts of thousands of caring and dedicated volunteers, donors, and host-country colleagues, Interplast has provided more than 35,000 free surgeries for people who might otherwise never have received the medical help they needed.

Interplast's Mission Statement

Interplast's mission is to provide free reconstructive surgery for people in developing nations, and to help improve health care worldwide. The organization's goals are to establish, develop, and maintain host-country, domestic-patient, and educational programs with the following objectives:

§ Provide direct patient care—reconstructive surgery and ancillary services to those with no other resources.

§ Provide educational training and medical interchange.

§ Assist host-country medical colleagues toward medical independence.

§ Enable recipients of care to become providers of care to new sites.

Interplast maintains no political or religious affiliations.

Sensitivity to, and respect for, other cultures as equals pervades the Interplast philosophy and deeply influences the manner in which we conduct ourselves as ambassadors.

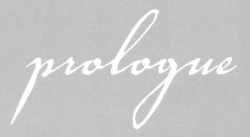

prologue

I RECEIVED MY SINGING VOICE AS A GIFT. WITH it I have attempted to tap into and touch the essence of human feelings, in their blackness and in their brilliance. Most of my life I've sung to entertain, to soothe, to bring laughter and tears to people from the privileged to the poverty stricken. And I've also used it to support causes dear to me. In doing so, I've inevitably received gifts in return.

When we see someone in need, like it or not, it is like holding a mirror up to ourselves, because the basic needs of life—food, human warmth, medical care, freedom, love, and acceptance—are universal needs. Since those needs are not universally met, I believe we are meant as a species to serve each other and to reach out to those who are isolated from us and society. And in that reaching out, in that service, we find that we ourselves are served.

The people who volunteer with and support Interplast participate in miracle-producing medical care that repairs a child's face and restores a family's spirit, giving back to them the life they were meant to have. The gratefulness of those healed, often from terrible malformations, is unbounded. They need no longer be the pariahs of their society. They may experience love and warmth for the first time. At the same time each person involved in Interplast's work will tell you that, no matter what the level of strain, exhaustion, sorrow, overwork, and frustration, his or her own life

will never be the same again. It, too, will be mysteriously transformed and immeasurably richer.

It has been my lifetime's experience that what we do to serve our fellow human beings is what gives us our own humanity.

May *The Gift* be a mirror for you.

Joan Baez
Woodside, California
July 2000

foreword

For the Love of Children
By Diane Ackerman

SAN PEDRO SULA SITS IN THE NORTHWEST CORNER of Honduras. On a tree-shaded street in the center of town stands the public hospital, a sprawling maze of one-story buildings, porticoes, and courtyards. Its corrugated roofs have grown rusty over the years, and the peeling walls are painted pink and maroon, with a ribbon of green, yellow, and red (the national colors) dancing at eye level. Outdoor benches, overflowing with patients and their families, sit on a checkerboard of yellow and green tiles. People fill the wards, crowd the walkways, and spill into the courtyards.

In the clinic waiting room, a hundred people sit back-to-back on long train-station benches. All are waiting to see the doctors of Interplast, an organization based in Mountain View, California, which sends out teams of medical volunteers to provide reconstructive surgery to needy children in the Third World.

A typical team includes three surgeons, four anesthesiologists, five nurses, a pediatrician, and a secretary. Housed with local families, a team works with their local counterparts, and high school students or other locals act as translators. When children need repairs that can't be done in their own country, they're sent to the United States as part of Interplast's domestic program.

IT IS ONLY 9:30 A.M. A THICK LINE OF PEOPLE winds among the benches. Parents have brought children with lost or malformed eyes, children with cleft lips and twisted feet, children with webbed hands, children with bad burns. Mingling with them are the success stories: children returning for touch-up operations, or to have their progress checked. Some families have been waiting for twenty-four hours, others have traveled great distances, on foot and by bus, from the mountains and the coast. Babies are being fed or changed; older children play or lie sleeping. Overhead, two large fans turn slowly, stirring but not cooling the hot, soupy air.

This is "Clinic Day" for the Interplast team, which flew in last night. Before the operations begin, the surgeons have to see the children, carefully examine their problems, and conduct a difficult triage. The sad truth is that someone with a defect requiring all day to do will have to be turned away, since a greater number of people could be helped in the same time. Eye surgery is also out, as well as anything else that could lead to massive complications. The hospital doesn't have the equipment, the cardiac facilities, or the supplies of blood and other necessities for a crisis, so they must choose reasonably healthy children, with defects operable under severely limited conditions.

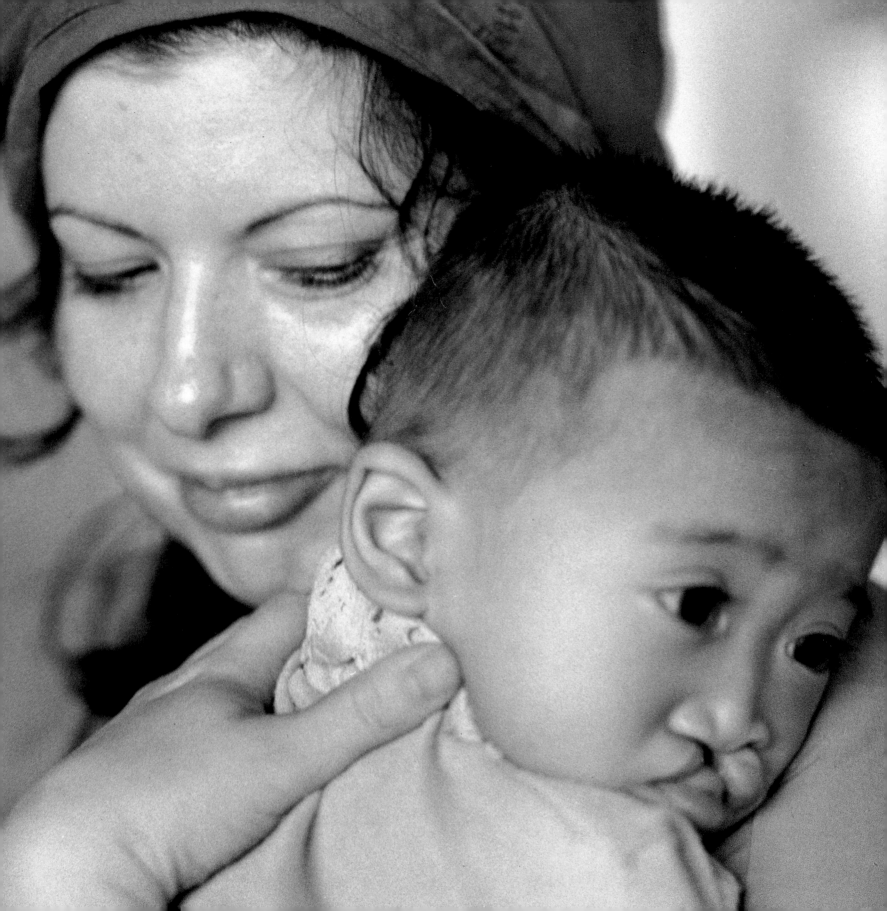

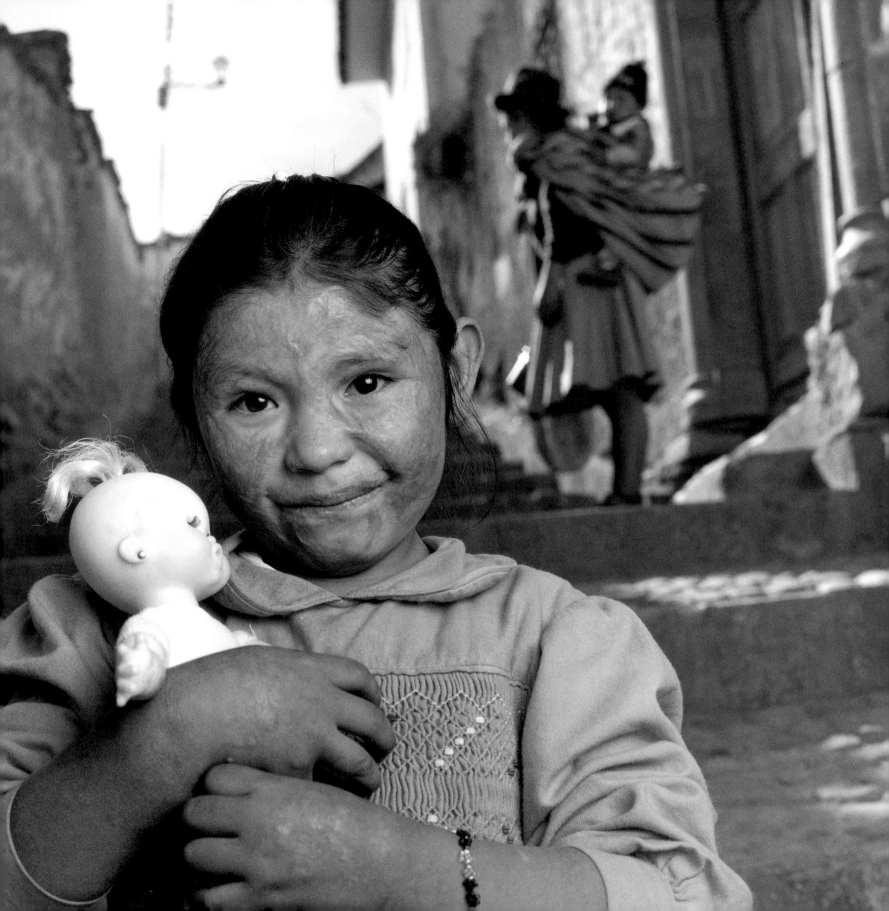

Although the team members have many reasons for making the trip, some purely altruistic, some more self-concerned, learning to *make do* with the minimum —indeed, discovering what that minimum is—is probably one of them. They will also have a chance to take part in tough, challenging operations they may only have read about; to do medicine the way it was done in the days before high technology; to improvise with few supplies and much cunning; to solve problems that, left untreated for too long, have become nightmarish and almost unsolvable, except through high-wire acts of virtuoso surgery; to learn techniques from others faced with the same rigors. That it will stir them deeply, and may prompt them to inspect their feelings about medicine, is also part of the draw. In a sense, it is a way to renew their vows.

In Room 9, surgeons Ruth Carr and Dean Sorensen sit behind two wooden desks, waiting for their first patients. Ruth is trim and petite with shoulder-length blond hair, wearing a denim skirt and a green shirt with a small pink polo player on the chest. She practices in Santa Monica and has a twenty-month-old son. This is her second Interplast trip. On her desk, a brown plastic pot of tongue depressors stands next to a purse-size flashlight—her only examination instruments. Across the room, behind the second desk, sits Sorensen, a tall, athletic, sandy-haired man, wearing a starched white coat over tan pants and a green shirt. Ruth speaks Spanish, but we also have in the room a teenage girl from the local international high school, who acts as an interpreter. Schoolmates of hers circulate throughout the other clinic rooms, translating, carrying Coca-Colas and files, and running errands.

A young mother enters, cradling a two-month-old girl named Isabel in her arms. Dean seats them on a stool beside his desk. Dressed in a blue shift, with a simple black cross on a black thread around her neck, the mother sits with the baby pressed snug against her shoulder and arranges the baby's bright red blouse, red socks, and diapers held by yellow-capped safety pins. Isabel's hair is a small cyclone of dark brown. The mother rocks her as she cries. "Why is the child here today?" Dean asks through the interpreter.

The mother turns her baby's face toward us, so we can see the completely cleft mouth and exposed nasal passages. It is a savagely disfiguring birth defect, in which the mouth appears to be split in two and turned partly inside out. Otherwise, she is a stunning little girl with loam-brown eyes and mocha skin. Because her cleft is so wide she won't be able to touch her tongue to the roof of her mouth to speak during the crucial language-learning years. Many of the children Interplast sees today will have equally severe clefts, a birth defect that strikes one in every 600 people. Because the United States has so large a population (270 million), and birth defects are operated on right away, people with clefts aren't as visible as they are in Honduras, whose population is only 4 million, and where inbreeding and malnutrition may be contributing factors. Dean peers into Isabel's mouth, using a flashlight and a tongue depressor, questions the mother about the child's general health, then takes her photograph, and at last jots down her name on a master sheet. She is an ideal candidate for surgery.

At the moment, Isabel is incapable of smiling, and that makes her helpless, vulnerable, and unarmed. Her life will be simpler if she can speak normally, but it would be a dreadful nightmare if she couldn't smile.

For an infant, a smile is the real human coin of the realm, as valuable to a Maori girl as it is to a boy from New Jersey. A child needs to be able to engage adults in a broad, open smile that can stop them in their tracks, elicit love, and turn antipathy to goodwill. Smiles are infectious, and rejuvenative. Adults find smiling, happy children more attractive, and attractive children receive more attention from teachers and more encouragement and affection from their parents. Smiling is an essential part of the shy pantomime we call flirting.

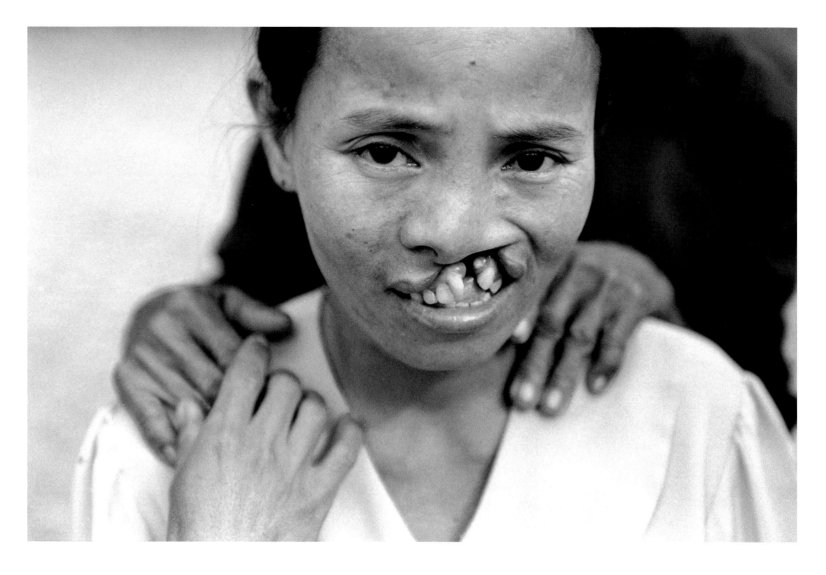

But a child also needs a normal mouth to perform that large repertoire of nonverbal signs we make with our faces, revealing moods according to a set pattern that people instinctively understand and expect. There is a code of basic facial expressions which all humans share—happiness, anger, fear, surprise, disgust—which are recognizable to people from different cultures, who speak different languages, who have never met, who seem to have nothing in common. A face is only bone, cartilage, tissue, and skin. And yet when these components work in unison as they were meant to, they create many thousands of subtle expressions. Children who are born blind make the same expressions as those who are sighted. Spontaneous, automatic, the face forms words before the mind can think them. We often rely on facial semaphore to tell us truths too subtle or shameful or awkward or intimate or emotionally charged or nameless to speak. Cancel that language of the smile and glance and you doom a child to a lifetime of emotional formality and effort, you cast it out of normal society.

ISABEL LEAVES, AND THE PARADE OF CHILDREN continues. By midafternoon, all the children begin to blur into one compound child, afflicted with itself, temporarily betrayed by its body. Many would profit from going to the United States for treatment, but Interplast can afford to send only twenty children a year, since it depends entirely on private donations of money, air tickets, and supplies. On principle, it has no government funding (and therefore no political interference), and the air tickets, especially, are expensive. So, instead, an Interplast doctor will often begin reconstructive work—to remove part of a burn scar, say, or do the first part of a cleft mouth-and-palate operation —on a child whom another Interplast doctor will continue operating on six months later.

This works out all right for the children, and it unites the surgeons in a powerful invisible chain. For, although the doctors who patrol the world for Interplast seldom meet face-to-face, they often meet in the body of a single child. In May, one doctor will operate on a cleft mouth; in September another will examine his predecessor's work and go on to do the palate; the following May yet another doctor will pick up the scalpel and perhaps fix a small hole in the roof of the mouth; the following September, another doctor may try to give the nose a longer and more natural philtrum. In this way, a child's life sentence is rewritten, over many months, by many hands, with sutures.

Cleft mouths are by far the most frequent deformity. According to the folklore of many countries, the "harelip" is a result of a pregnant mother being frightened by a rabbit. This was so widespread a belief in Europe that an old Norwegian law actually forbade butchers from hanging up rabbits in public view. It was always the mother's evil, sin, or contract with the Devil for which the deformed child was a punishment. During the Middle Ages, if a child's deformity looked in any way animal-like it was concluded that the mother had had sex with the animal, and the deformed child was their offspring. Such children were killed. So, fixing a child's cleft lip also, in part, repairs the supernatural burdens of a family.

BY 6:00 P.M. THE WAITING ROOM HOLDS ONLY A few adults, the clinic rooms have grown dimmer. In this room alone, Ruth and Dean have examined eighty patients. "It's a bottomless well," Ruth says, leaning wearily against the wall.

Operations begin the next morning. Swinging doors open onto a small room, glared over by exposed fluorescent lights, where two operating tables stand parallel, about ten feet apart. The blue tile walls give way to green paint at shoulder level, and the olive-green tiled floors look ready for a track meet.

The three operating rooms are over eighty years old, and one of them has an opaque wall of glass bricks. A few years ago, when the electricity failed during an evening operation, Luis Bueso, who heads the project in Honduras, ran outside and pointed his car's headlights at the glass wall, and nurses held flashlights above the operating tables.

As the morning gives way to the afternoon and early evening, Spanish, French, Portuguese, and English mix in the operating rooms, where a procession of children arrive from their villages, appear suddenly on the tables, have their faces and lives rearranged while they are unconscious, and disappear into the recovery room and then into the pediatrics ward. Not only the children dwell in this shudder out of time. All of us are temporarily yanked out of the normal course of our lives. Teams are thrown together in emotionally charged circumstances, and, as a result, people often form intense friendships and interdependencies. Then the red alert of the trip ends suddenly, like a small death, and, returning home, team members often sink into parabolas of depression.

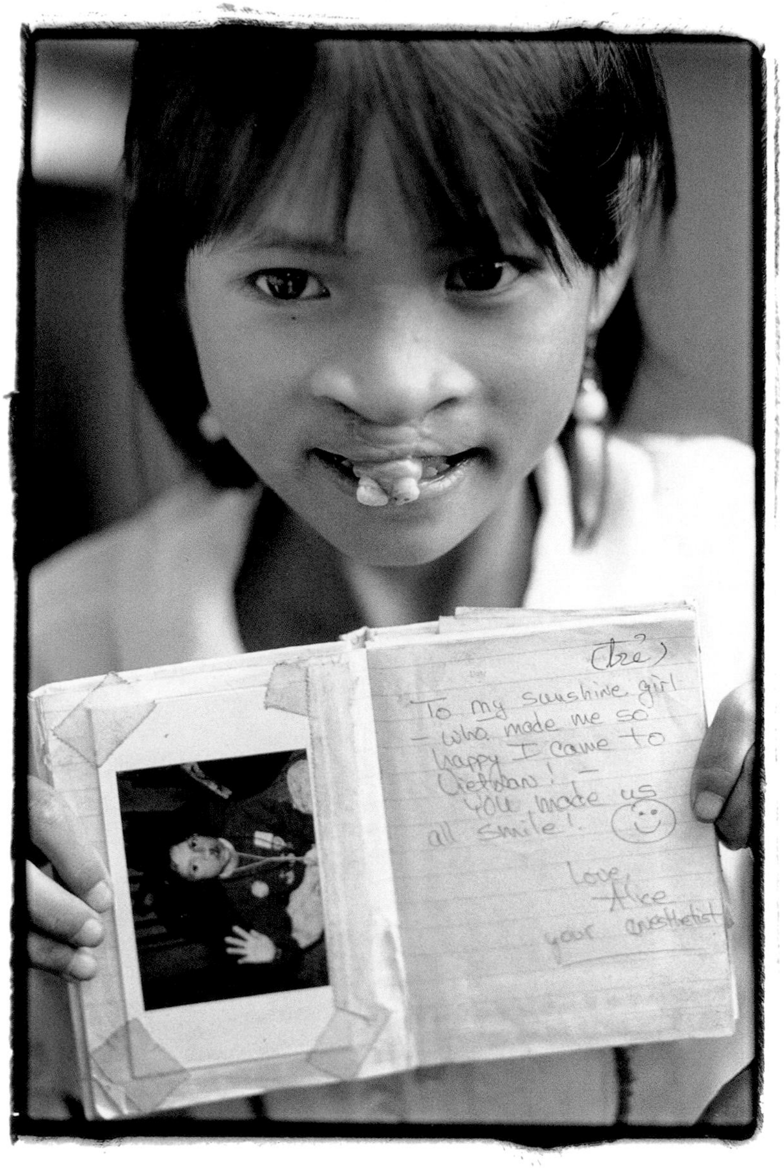
To my sunshine girl
— who made me so
happy I came to
Vietnam! —
You made us
all smile!
Love,
Alice
your anesthetist

"It's strange not knowing the before and after," surgeon Dave Thomas says. "Suddenly these children appear with their predicaments. Then they vanish. You only see them at that one moment in time. In that moment, you may be changing the whole course of their lives. But you never see them again. The good part is that plastic surgery is unique in that, with many surgeries—a hernia, for example—you can't see the result right away. But I can see right away what I've done to reconstruct an arm or, especially, a face."

By midweek, there are signs of our presence on all the children: colored deputy sheriff badges, colored barrettes and earrings, toy trucks and tops and puzzles, new dresses and T-shirts. In the children's ward, rows of full beds and cribs line the room. On one wall, a framed, yellowing picture of a Gerber baby's smiling and perfect face is the center of a large, open, dewy red rose. A hand-drawn rabbit with a merry smile and long lashes watches from the wall, near Raggedy Ann and Andy clothes hooks.

Although the hospital is old and worn, it is very clean, and it is staffed by a caravan of devoted nurses. They get paid little—indeed, sometimes don't get paid for weeks—yet they keep coming to work. In the same blue dress she wore to the clinic, Isabel's mother feeds her daughter with an eyedropper. Shaped normally now, her mouth wears a design of fine stitches. Cardboard splints on her arms will keep her from pestering the stitches until they dissolve. Whenever possible, the doctors use dissolvable stitches because they can't rely on the compliance of the patients, who might not have enough money to make a return trip. Mother bundles Isabel up in her arms, hugs her close. Smiling, relieved, she says good-bye and thanks everyone, emotionally, then turns around and thanks them all over again.

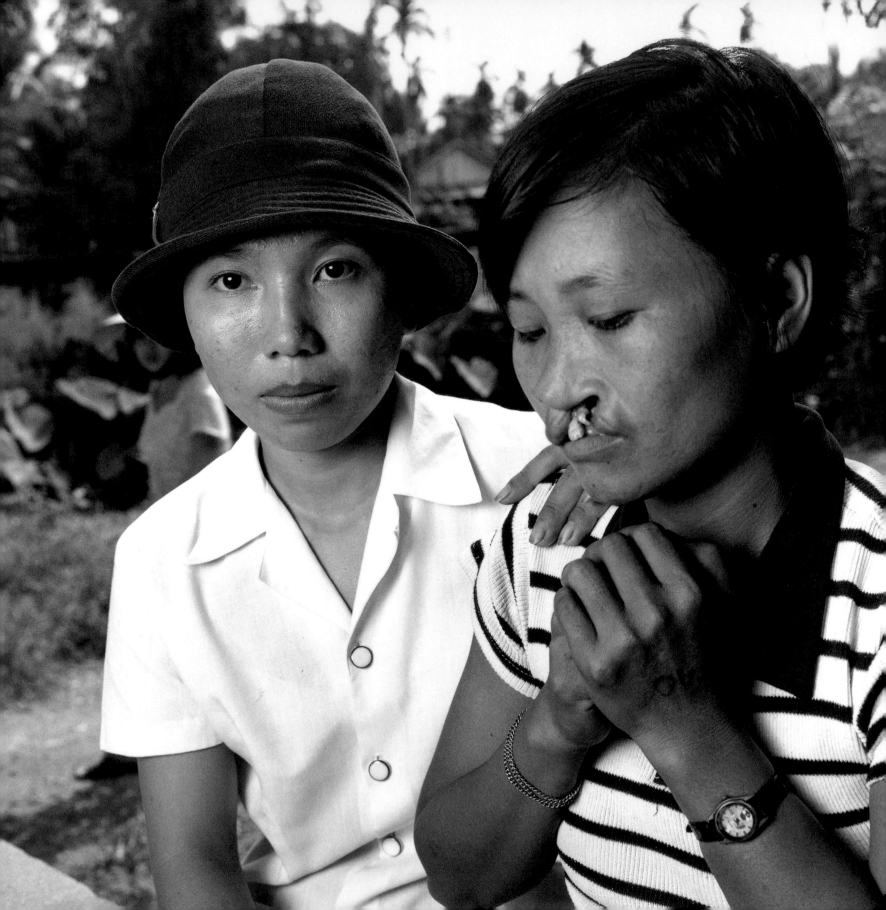

introduction

SEVERAL YEARS AGO, WHILE TREKKING IN A RE-
mote valley high in the Peruvian Andes, I came across
a Quechua family with a four-year-old girl who bore
a faint scar on her upper lip, very recognizable to me
as a cleft lip that had been surgically repaired.

The family insisted that I spend the night with
them in their one-room stone hut. They made every
attempt to treat me like royalty. When I inquired about
the scar, they told me that American doctors had come
to their country and had fixed the terrible deformity
their daughter had been born with. They couldn't thank
me enough.

A little over a year ago, I was asked by Interplast
if I would help create a book that would illustrate the
work they perform on children with facial deformities
who live in remote areas around the world. The project
called to me in several ways. First, I had traveled to
many of the areas they served. Secondly, as an ortho-
dontist I had worked in conjunction with oral surgeons
and plastic surgeons to treat patients with cleft palate
deformities in my practice for over eighteen years.

In all that time, I never saw a patient with an un-
operated cleft lip. In the developed world, infants with
cleft lips almost always have the problem corrected
within the first year of life. Not so in other parts of the
world, where this abnormality often remains uncor-
rected into adulthood and throughout life.

From a small child's perspective, a cleft is neutral;
however, there comes a day when that outward disfig-
urement begins to disfigure the spirit and psyche as
well. This pain of image, reputation, and self-worth

transcends culture. In Vietnam, it is believed that if a
pregnant woman merely looks at someone with a cleft,
her unborn baby will catch the affliction. In Peru, a
baby born with a congenital facial abnormality is considered to be the result of a previous sin of the mother.
It takes little imagination to recognize how deep the
pain can be for the whole family.

The photographs in this book—documenting two
trips taken by Interplast teams, one to Cuzco, Peru,
and one to Quang Ngai and Hoi An, Vietnam—are of
people in various stages of that pain. For infant José
Luis, the psychic pain has yet to begin. Hoi and Isabel,
schoolgirls an ocean apart, are united by their position
in that cycle of pain. Isabel's schoolmates call her a
monster. At seventeen, Bay is in the thick of life, ask-
ing existential questions. Lan, twenty-two years old,
with her aging mother literally her single friend on
earth, is reaching a state of resignation.

This book is also about those men and women
who perform procedures to heal that pain, and the
organization that unites the healers and the misshapen.
Finally, it is about the gift both receive as that process
takes its course.

The gift to the patient is obvious. But many of
these volunteers, who have it all, relatively speaking,
are surprised at what they come away with—much
deeper gifts. They told me about the gratitude they
receive—and about simply being able to do what
they're trained to do in an unencumbered way, without
the heavy overlay of bureaucratic rules; about the satisfaction of taking somebody whose facial features are

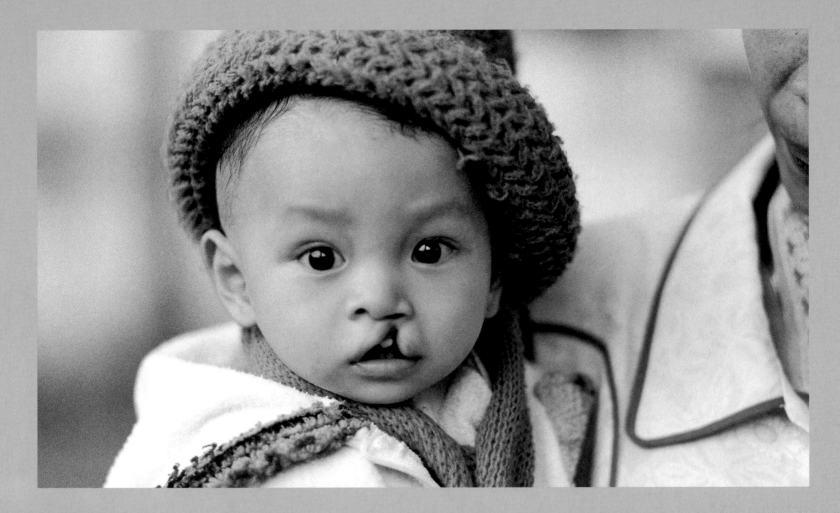

radically deformed and making them look pretty normal almost immediately.

However, it was the unanticipated recognition of what has slipped away—in their own culture, in their own profession, in their own lives—that became a deeper gift of perspective. For many, this image of loss became the enduring one. They saw the poise of the patients and their extended families, the time people spent with and for each other, the support perfect strangers gave to one another. These things that the volunteers noticed are values our culture has somewhat lost. They saw firsthand people content in the midst of relative hardship, and they came to realize the tendency toward personal isolation in the comfort of industrialized luxury.

And so, in the end, the gift is perspective. To say that everyone receives it would be to grossly romanticize. Nonetheless, perspective seems to be one of the broad, deep themes of an Interplast trip, and when the medical teams go home they leave with gratitude from their patients—and with renewed gratitude for their own lives.

The plastic surgery made possible worldwide by Interplast is relatively simple and enormously practical. The volunteers go off for two weeks, transform a hundred or more lives, return—and in so doing carry home the seeds of their own transformation.

Phil Borges
Seattle, Washington
July 1999

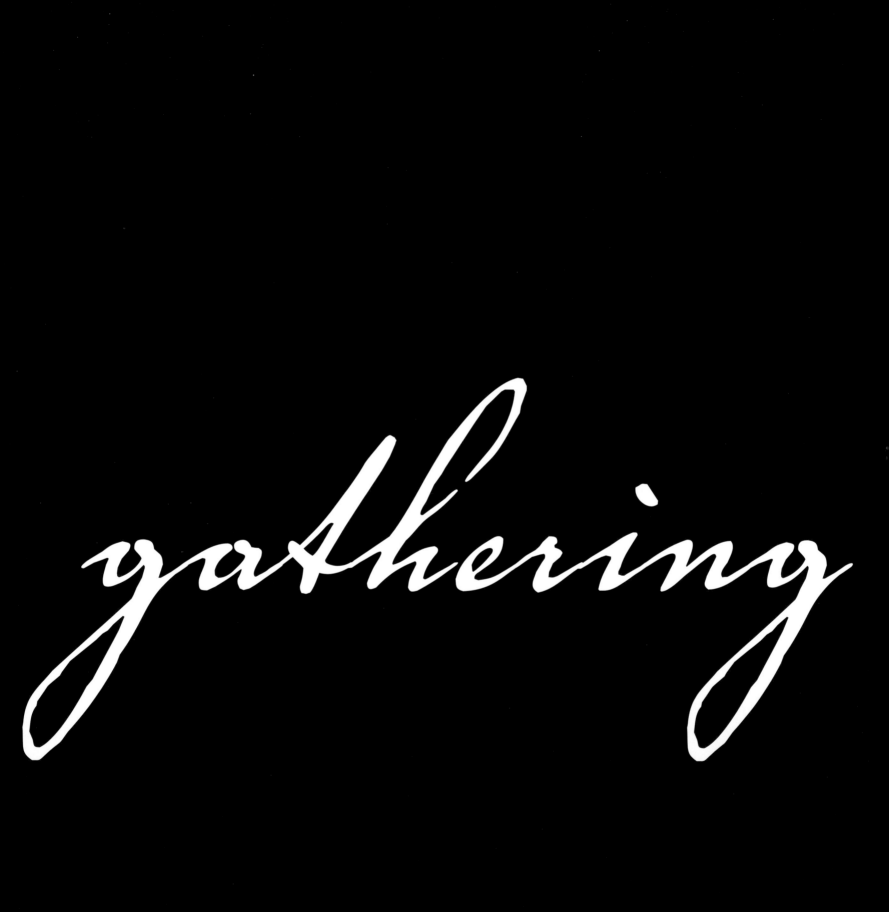

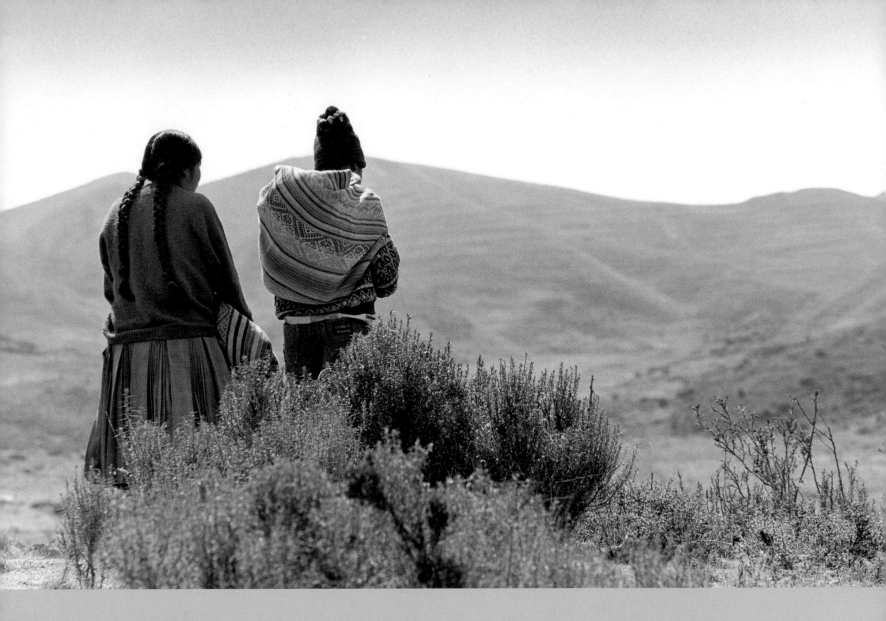

THE TEAM THAT TRAVELED TO PERU FIRST LINKED
up at the Dallas–Fort Worth airport: fourteen people
including surgeons, anesthesiologists, nurses, a pediatrician, and a secretary/interpreter. During the long
flight to Lima, the team was animated, getting to know
one another and discussing the upcoming events.

By the time they boarded the ninety-minute flight
from Lima to Cuzco, however, the team members had
grown subdued. They were tired and jet-lagged—a
few had been traveling for more than twenty-four hours
from their homes—and also reflective. Gazing out at

the Andes below, they saw only an occasional adobe
hacienda, its rock walls sculpted from the flank of a
mountainside, with perhaps a couple of sheep the only
living things visible and no other civilization for miles.
*Are the people we are going to treat coming from one of
these houses?*

A hospital representative greeted the group at the
gate in Cuzco and expedited customs. The equipment—
a half-ton of supplies in twenty large vinyl crates—
would follow on a later flight. The team didn't know
it at the time, but this equipment would be delayed for

*A Quechua family beginning the
trek to Cuzco.*

21

an entire week due to problems with the airline and customs.

Cuzco is a town of 200,000, some 12,000 feet above sea level. It has in recent years become a popular tourist destination, with good reason: it was the original capital and has a long history, a beautiful square, and buildings that have foundations dating from Inca times more than a thousand years ago. But the town's only hospital is far from the city center, the lovely plaza, and the other tourist destinations; it lies in a drab, more prosaic neighborhood on the fringes of town.

In the muted haze of the early morning, the team boarded a small bus and wound its way toward the Hospital Regional Cuzco, the sounds of roosters and car horns penetrating the bus windows. Everyone was a little tense; in particular, the faces of the first-time volunteers revealed a mixture of excitement and apprehension about performing their jobs in settings that lacked the ordinary amenities normally at their disposal.

An eight-foot iron fence surrounded the perimeter of the hospital, a five-story concrete structure resembling a warehouse from the outside. A guard waved the team members through; entering through the rear

On the way to the Cuzco hospital.

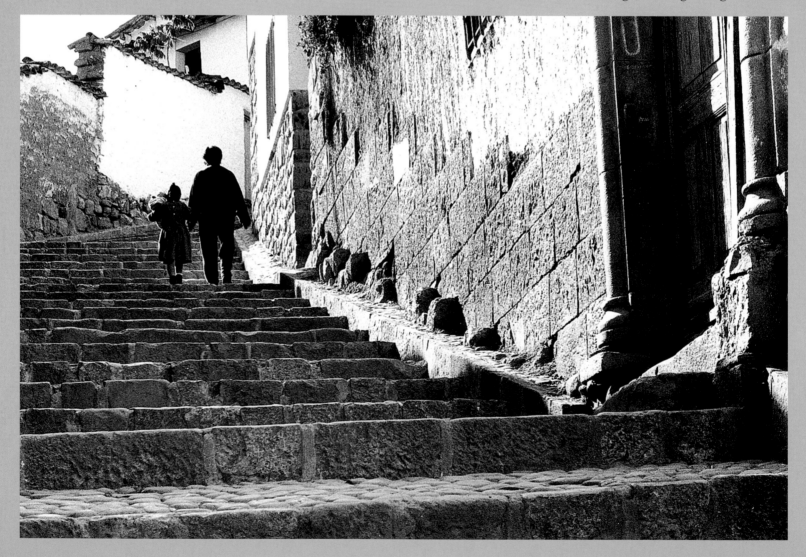

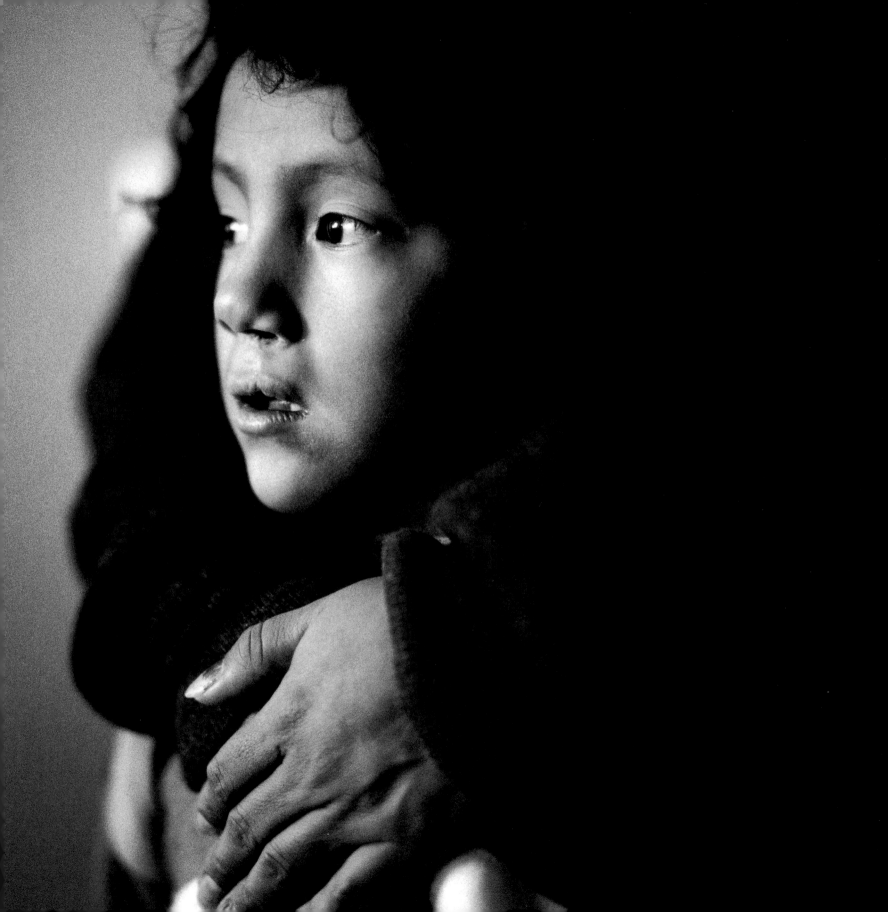

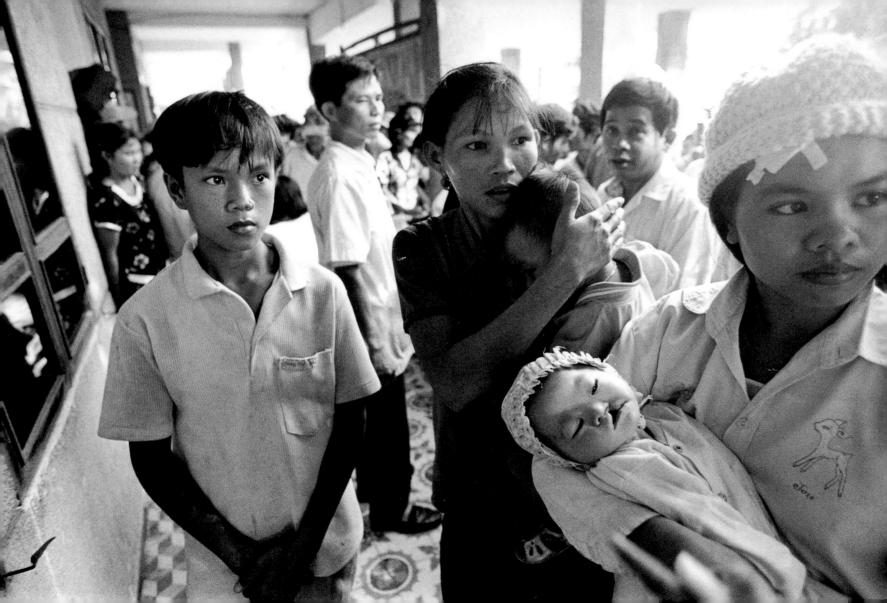

emergency-room door, they encountered a lobby bare except for a few metal folding chairs and a pair of men, waiting patiently with bandaged heads.

The entire top-floor ward had been emptied in preparation for the foreign guests. There was precious little time to relax, however. Everyone immediately washed up, donned white hospital coats and stethoscopes, and headed back down to begin the screening.

As the elevator doors opened into the clinic waiting room, a crowd of over two hundred broke into applause. Perhaps one in three wore the traditional woven blankets of the Quechua Indians. Many had been waiting there for days. Another, even larger, mass of people was visible outside the perimeter gates. They had come to the hospital from miles around, after hearing radio announcements and word of mouth that had radiated out of the city for weeks.

The throng rolled toward the medical team— whole families, including grandparents, babies, young children—enveloping them and speaking Spanish and Quechua as if everyone understood. *One moment, one moment, one moment, the interpreter's coming*. People displayed their babies, and their own burns and clefts —but smiling and clapping all the while.

And with the crowd came the rumbling mantra that Interplast volunteers hear over and over, in many situations and in many languages: *Dios le Paga, Dios le Paga, Dios le Paga*. Literally, this is *God Pays You*, but it carries the subtle, added poignancy of *God Will Repay You*.

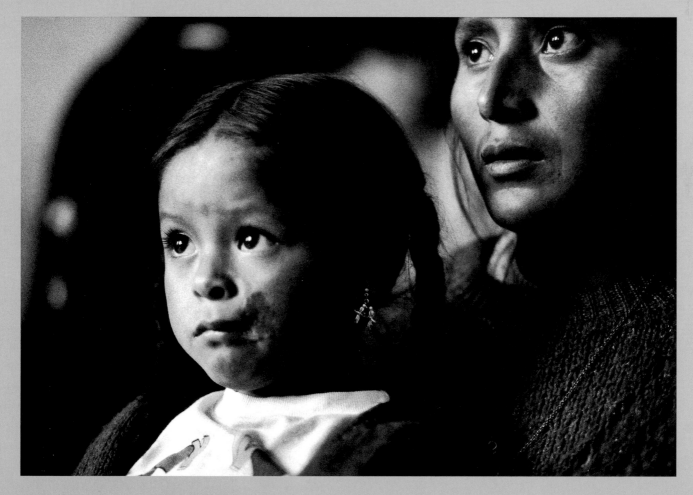

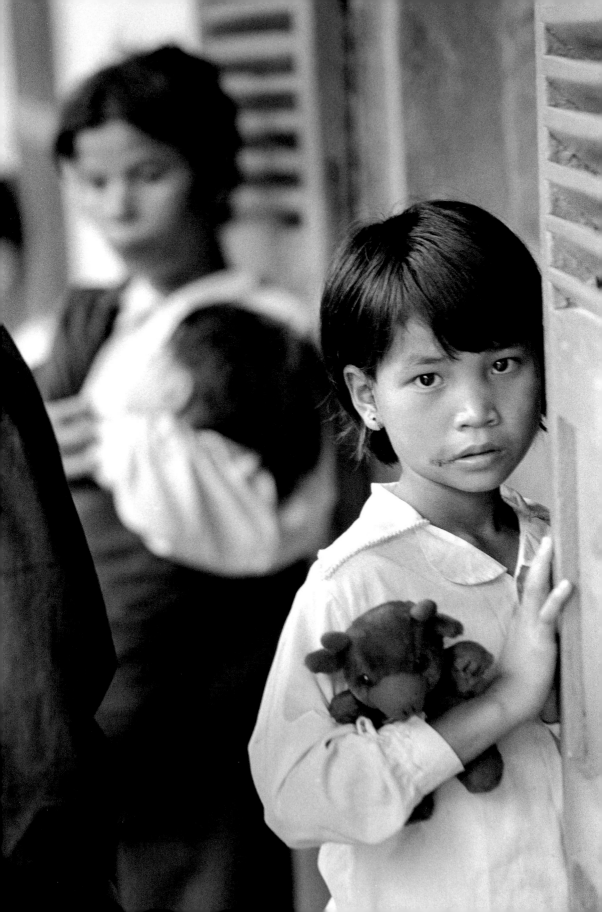

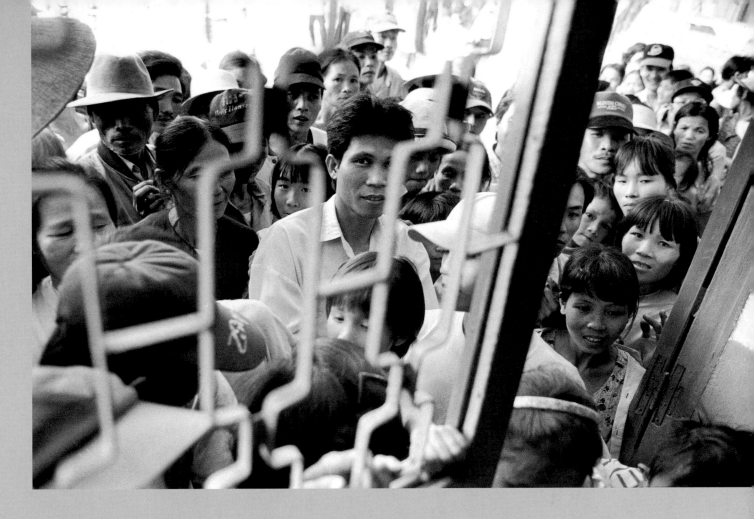

IN A SETTING AN OCEAN AWAY FROM PERU, Interplast had already made dozens of trips to Vietnam. But it was only in the last few years of the 1990s that it began working in Quang Ngai. The visible, outward emotion was less strong in Vietnam than in Peru, but underlying emotional currents struck the Vietnam team no less powerfully. The apprehensions there were of a different sort: the tangled, harsh history that separates Vietnam and the United States.

There was a particular poignancy to the destination. Quang Ngai lies close to the scene of perhaps the most notorious American tragedy in Vietnam: the My Lai massacre. The mother of one patient, Lan, lived only two kilometers from My Lai. She heard the shooting, saw the smoke from the burning huts, was forced to hide. Lan was born a few years later. No scientific evidence conclusively indicates this, but Lan's mother believed, as many Vietnamese do, that her daughter's monstrously deformed mouth and jumble of teeth were caused by Americans dumping the chemical defoliant Agent Orange out of the sky.

The irony of this new situation—an American team flying back in, twenty-five years later, with another kind of payload—was hardly subtle. How would Interplast be received?

But My Lai never came up. In fact, the war was never mentioned by any of the Vietnamese, to the amazement of the medical team. They encountered only gratitude, trust, and the surprising faith patients and their families had in a group of white-coated strangers from a country that had once fought on their soil.

Hospital entrance, Day one, Hoi An.

screening

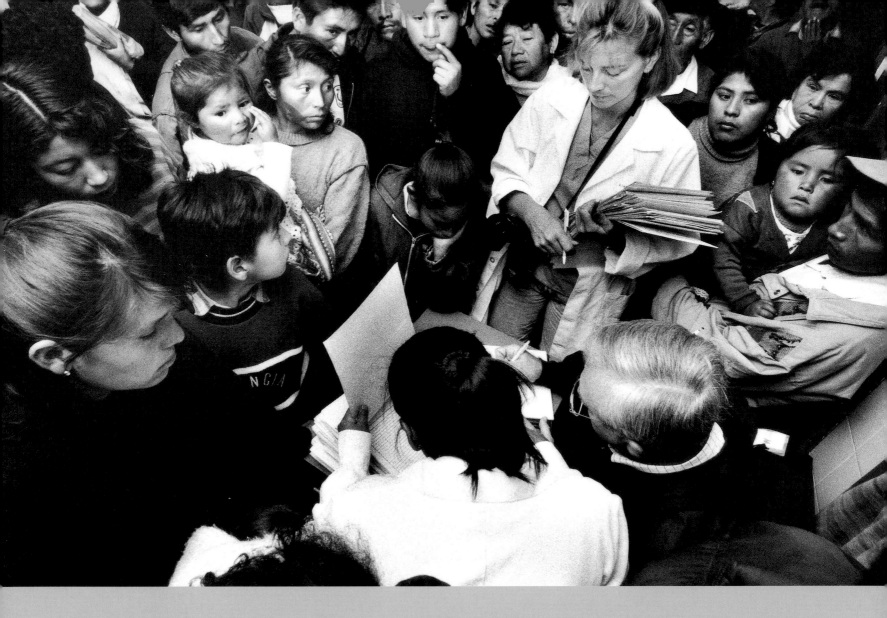

Initial sign-in, Cuzco.

IN BOTH PERU AND VIETNAM, MANY POTENTIAL patients had already been prescreened by local physicians before the arrival of the teams. Of these, the Interplast teams would screen, in each instance, roughly two hundred patients over the course of the first few days.

The process in Peru began for the team when its secretary, a fluent Spanish speaker, was given a list by a hospital official. The crowd that pressed around him formed no lines. It was a big, amorphous mass, and yet there was virtually no pushing or shoving. It became eerily quiet as Steve called out a name. Then a wave of murmurs would ripple through the assembly.

If the person called out wasn't present, the motion of the crowd let you know: others would fan out, calling the name. Presently someone would be propelled forward—often a little kid on total alert, wide-eyed with fascination and shock—and be ushered along with family members into the screening room.

You could hear them thinking: *Is this the operation?* Their equilibrium was upset; they had no idea what was about to happen. But stoic. Everybody remarked

29

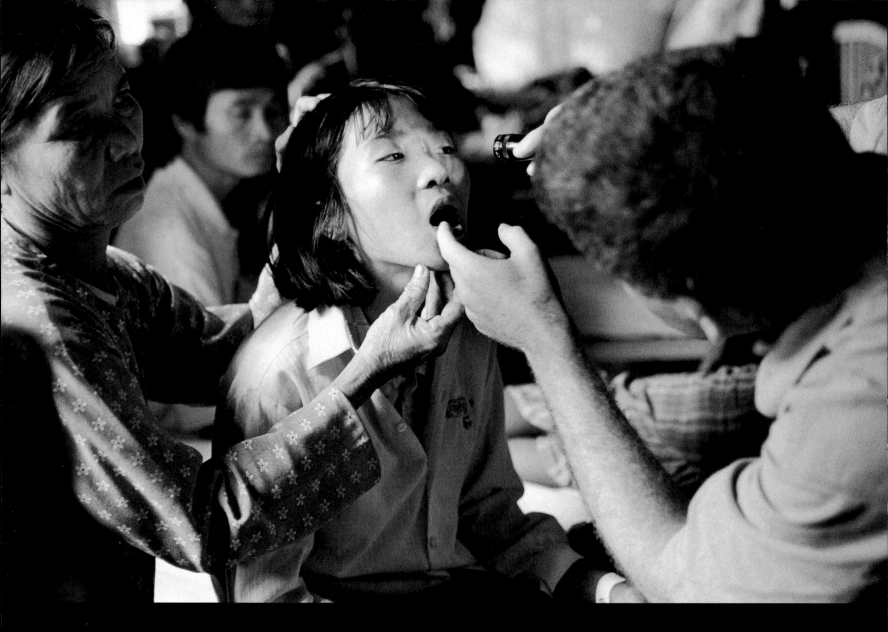

Screening a cleft-palate patient,
Quang Ngai.

These people come from such distances, under such hardships, and they were
so patient. That first morning when we walked in and it was mobbed—it
was just wall-to-wall people . . . and they saw us approaching and they broke
into applause. I don't know when I have had anything touch me so. To know
these people came from so far, believing we were the ones who could help
their children—I've never had a feeling like that before.

—Barbara

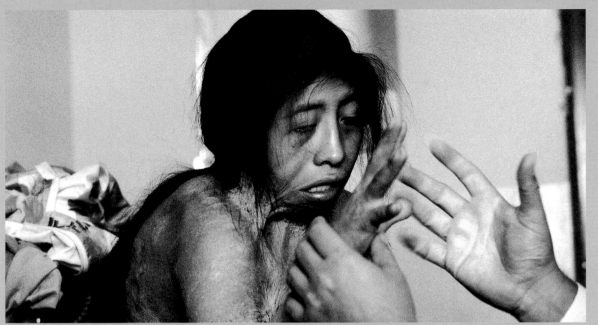

Screening burn patient, Cuzco.

about that sense of stoicism, not just in Peru but in Vietnam. It was replayed when patients entered surgery: four-year-olds walking into an operating room, surrounded by masked strangers who spoke an alien language. Often they'd hop up onto the table and help hold their anesthesia masks, never having even seen an anesthesia mask, murmuring *gracias* or *cam on* as they went under.

There were heartbreaking exceptions. Maybe one in fifteen people were turned away, told they couldn't be helped, because the baby had bronchitis or a simple cold or some other condition that would preclude surgery; children with a respiratory condition cannot be anesthetized safely. It was devastating to tell a mother who has walked God knows how far, hope building every step of the way, that *No, we can't help your child because he has this cough*. The best the team could say was that they would probably be back the next year.

As the screening went on, the next steps were already beginning. Patients and their families would leave the crowd around the secretary only to find another crowd in the screening room. There might be three patients in that room at a time. A surgeon was examining the first, with a nurse taking notes. A pediatrician was seeing a second, checking for colds or anything else that might prevent safe anesthesia. A scheduler worked with the third patient, providing an appointment day and a number, written on the chest with indelible ink. The number went on, the patient left, and outside another name would be called out, repeating the process.

Interplast doctors and nurses cannot afford to wait around and perform only the specialized jobs they normally perform. The focus is strictly on the medicine, on getting the job done. In Vietnam, for instance, while some of the volunteers screened patients, the anesthesiologists were busy setting up the operating room, not normally their job. In Peru, while waiting for the way-laid equipment, the team did what it could; for example, the anesthesiologists were involved in the screening process, helping the nurses and pediatricians assemble information. Thanks to this cooperation, their common goal—getting the job done—was already helping groups of strangers to become close-knit teams.

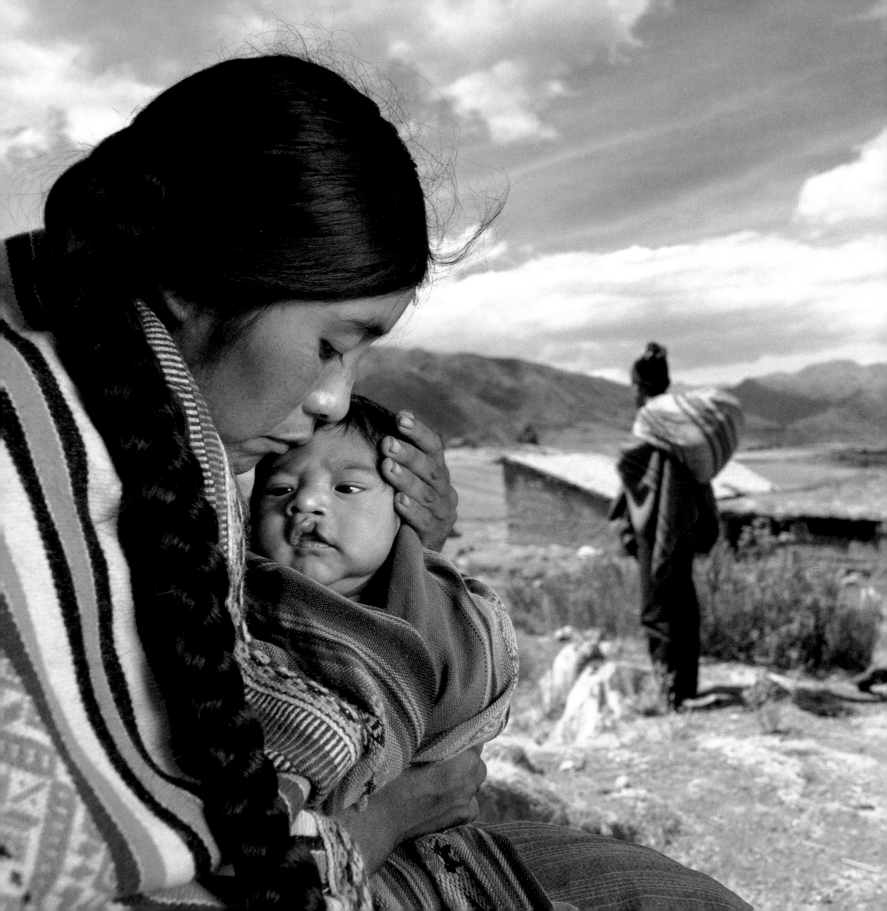

josé luis

Like most children in his Peruvian village, José Luis was born on the dirt floor of his parents' one-room adobe hut. José Luis was their first child.

His young mother, Leonardia, was terrified when she first noticed his facial deformity. Because of a prevalent Quechua belief that such deformities are somehow related to the sins of the mother, Leonardia carried a strong sense of personal guilt along with the sadness she felt for her baby.

Five weeks after José Luis's birth, his father, Alario, was working in his field when a neighbor told him that a medical team might be coming to Cuzco. The neighbor had heard that the team was able to correct facial birth defects.

Alario ran home and told Leonardia the news. The next morning they began the fifty-mile trek to Cuzco, partly along small footpaths through tiny villages until they could reach a bus line. Five days later, their baby's lip repaired, they were returning to their home high in the Andes.

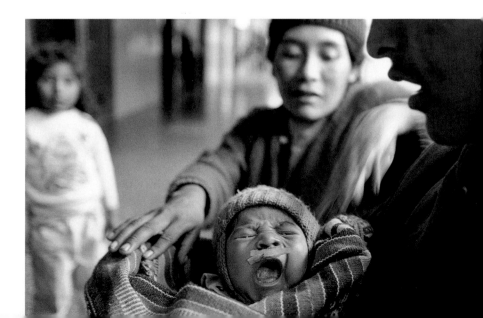

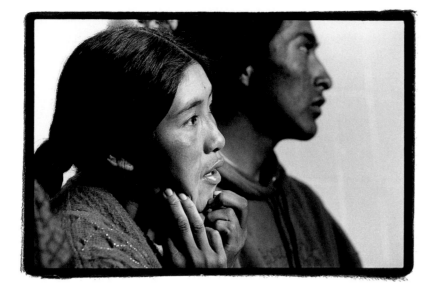 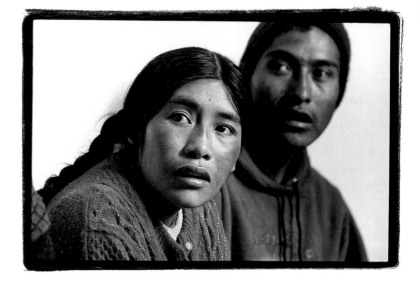

It was hard to read the look of these parents—their faces crossed the line between hope and uncertainty. They'd never even been in a hospital before, but they entrusted their most precious possession—a five-week-old baby—to these strangers with whom they couldn't even communicate.

—*Phil Borges*

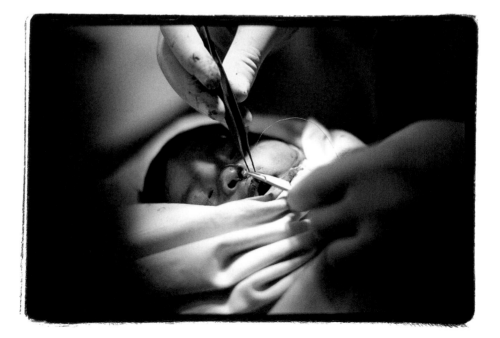

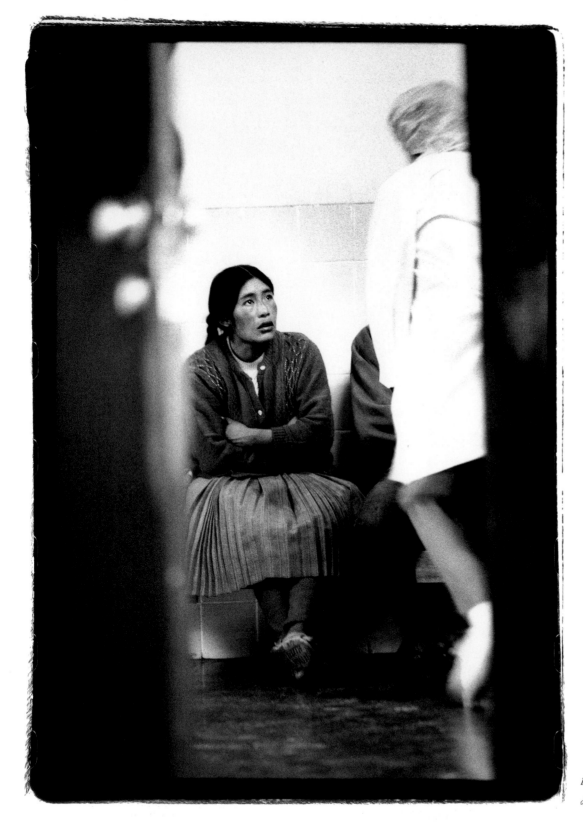

Reassuring José Luis's parents

during the operation.

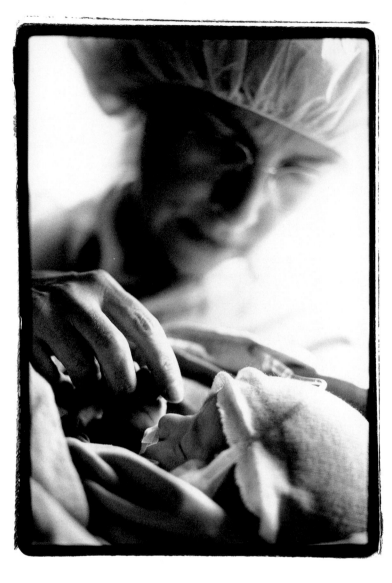

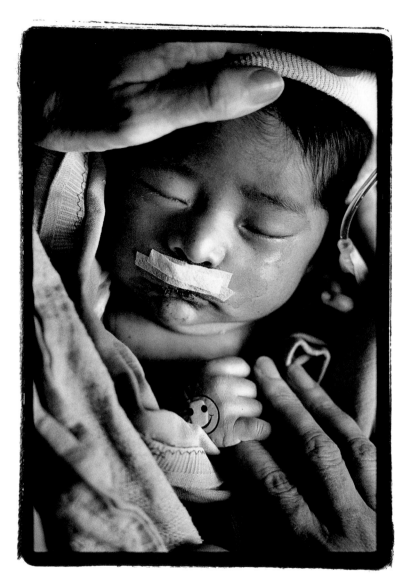

Preparing José Luis for his mother's first look.

We decided to let the parents in the recovery room. They were so anxious to see their kids that we just put them in scrubs and brought them in. We don't usually do this in the States, but I just felt it was important.

—*Barbara*
RECOVERY ROOM NURSE
SALT LAKE CITY, UTAH

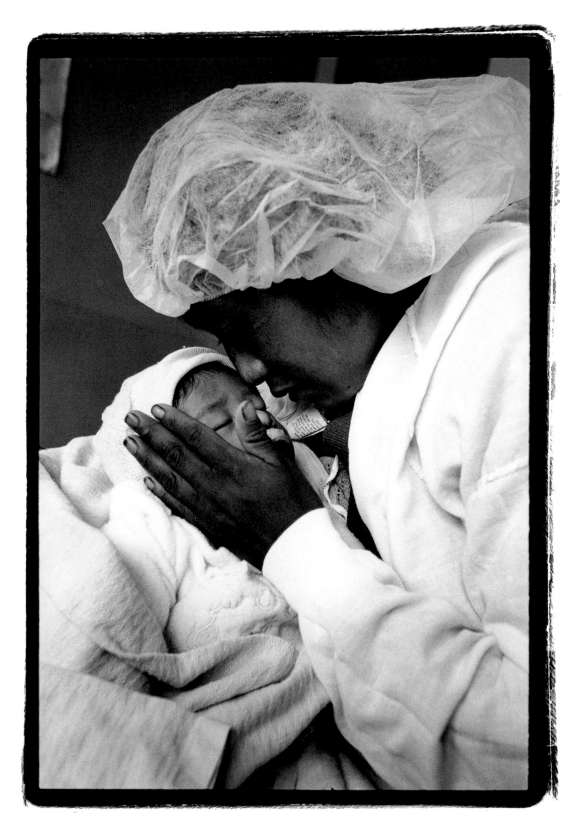

José Luis has been in the recovery room just long enough to get a lot of the anesthesia out of his system and begin waking up. His mother has been brought in and given her baby, and she just gets lost. She tries to feed her baby immediately. She just wants to get back into that role of mothering José.

—*Maureen*

RECOVERY ROOM NURSE

BERKELEY, CALIFORNIA

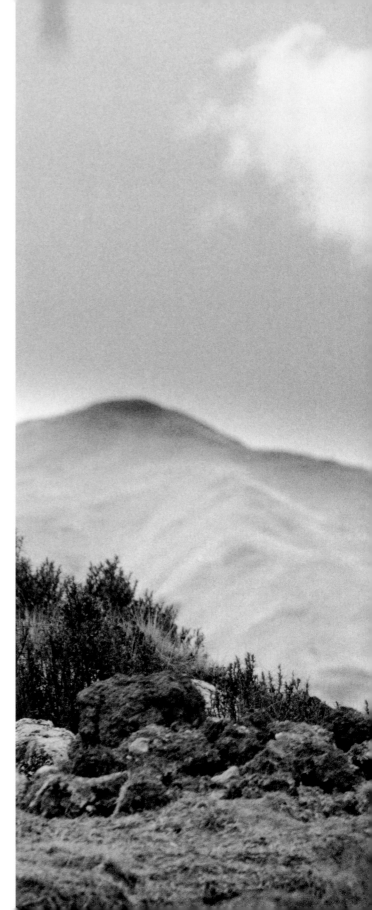

Returning home.

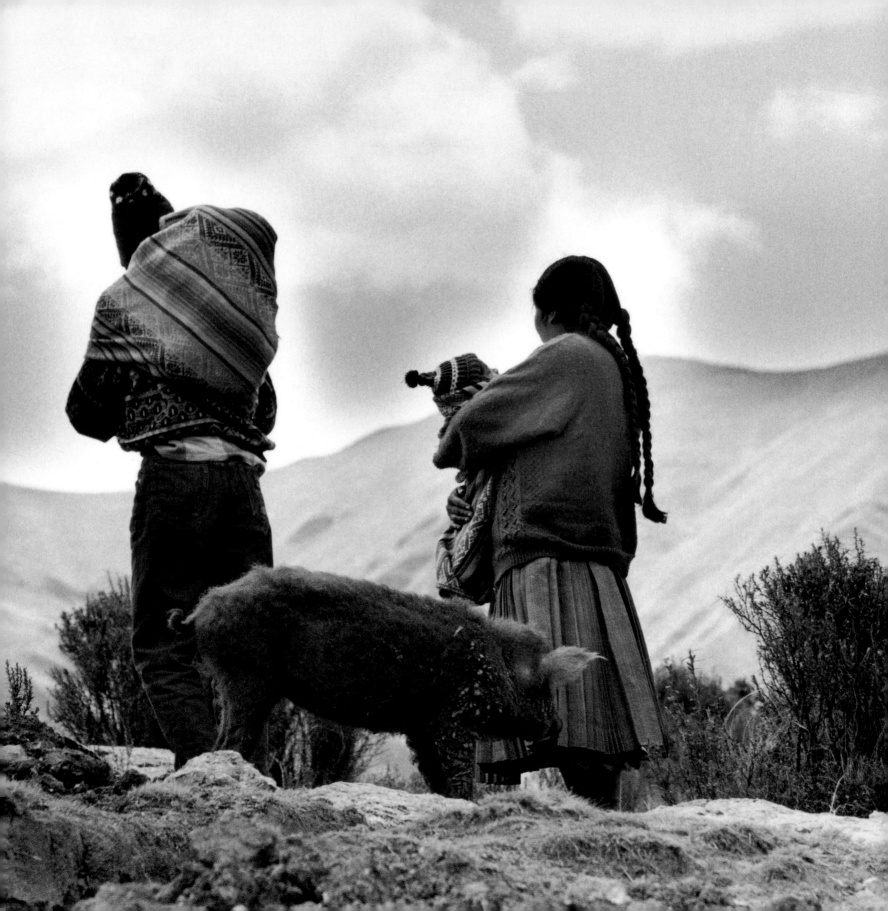

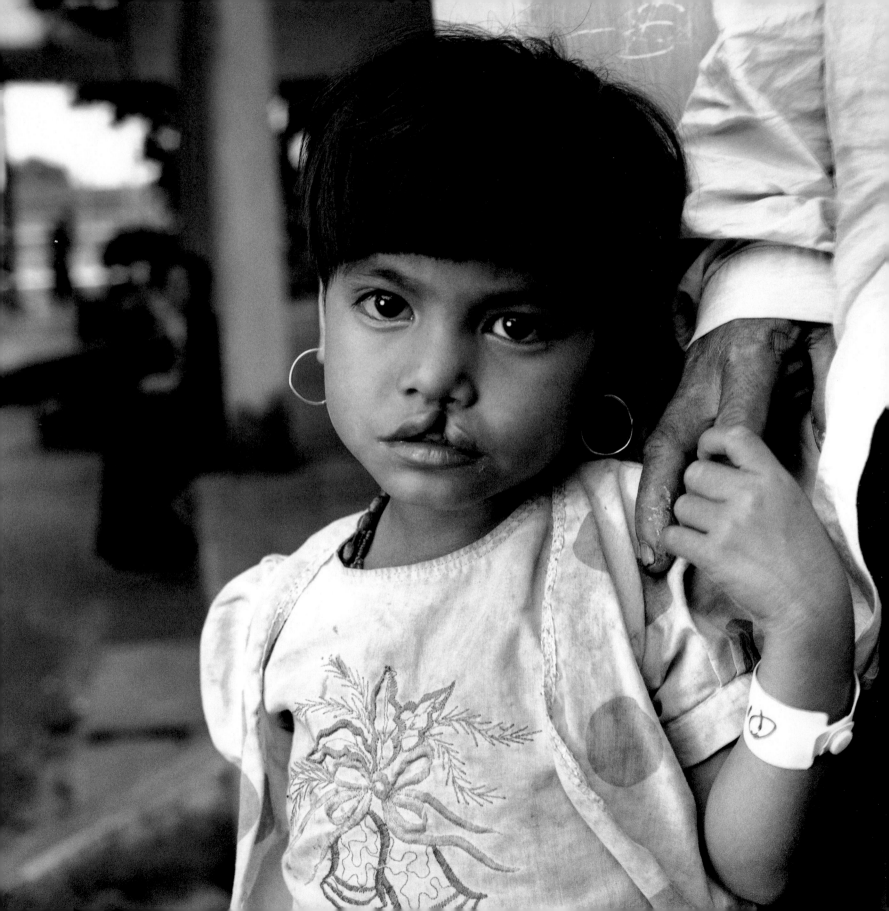

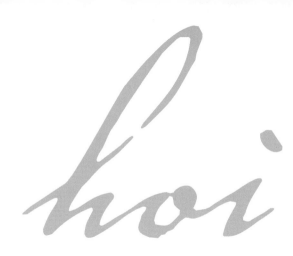

hoi

Hoi belongs to the Re village in Vietnam's central highlands.

The tribe raises corn and rice and hunts wild animals in order to survive; nonetheless, they are very close to extinction. There are, in fact, only ten families left.

Nan, Hoi's mother, heard about Interplast through a friend who heard it on the radio. Although she was very nervous about coming to the "city," Nan walked nearly thirty-five miles out of the mountains to catch the bus to Quang Ngai.

Nan's village was bombed several times during the war. She believes her daughter's condition was caused by Agent Orange, the chemical defoliant used by the U.S. military in Vietnam. Many Vietnamese share this belief, although no scientific studies have proved or disproved the theory.

When it was time for Hoi to be taken into surgery, Nan could not let her go. She held onto Hoi tightly and shivered for quite a while. When Nan was finally able to let her daughter go she said, "I believe in what the Americans can do." Hoi's surgery was completed in less than thirty minutes.

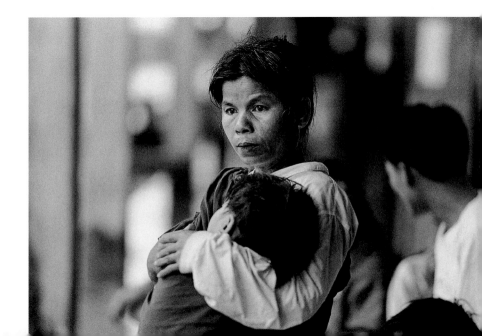

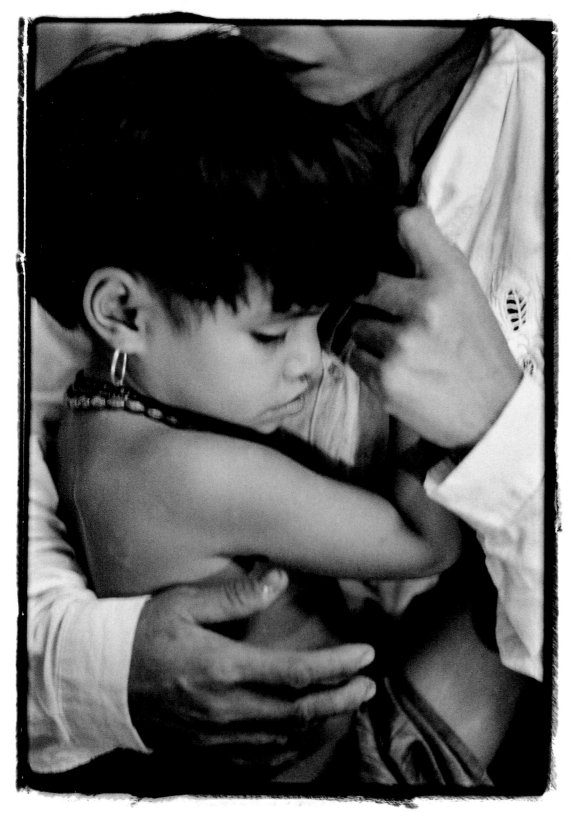

Since she was from a mountain tribe, there was no one who could speak with Hoi's mother. I noticed her uncertainty from the very beginning: Am I doing the right thing? Can I trust these people? When the moment arrived to hand Hoi over, she clung to her child and trembled for a full five minutes. Eventually, she regained her composure and was able to give Hoi to the nurse.

—Phil Borges

Hoi cradled in her mother's arms.

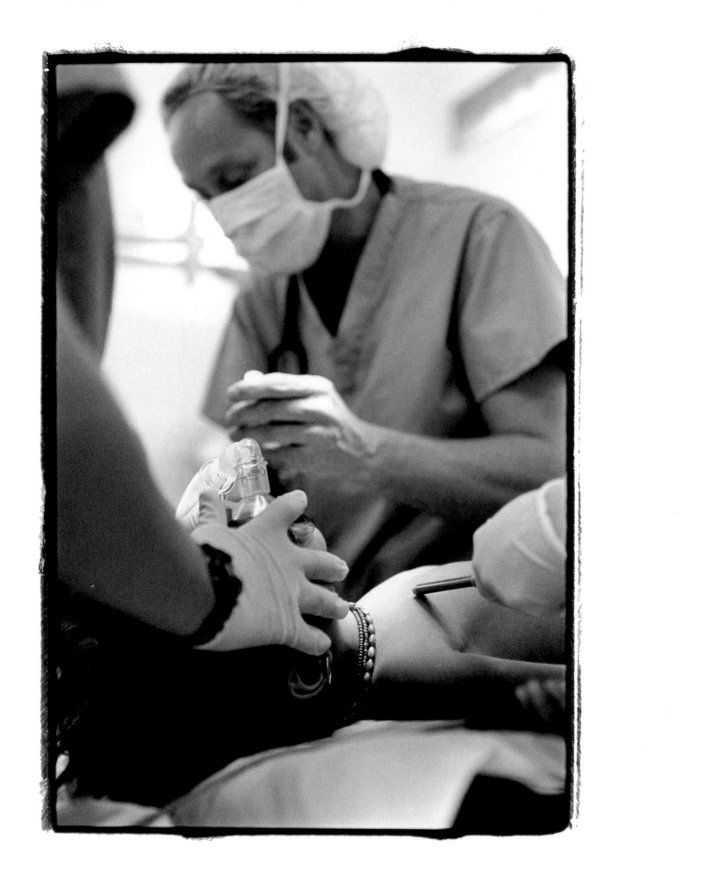

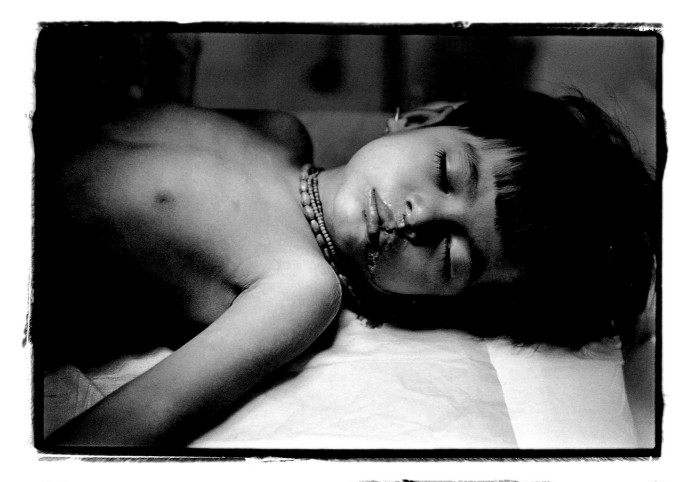

Hoi in the recovery room.

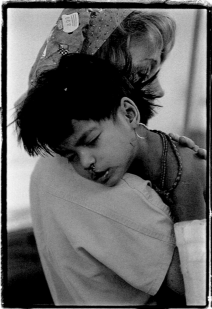

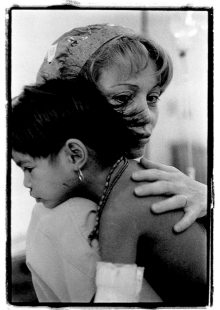

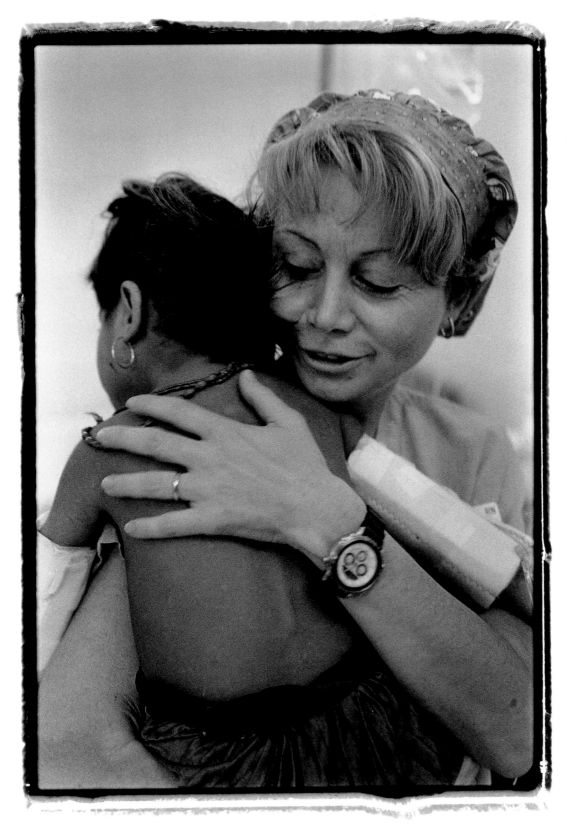

I've been on Interplast trips to Central and South America before, and there the mothers are just so emotional when they see their babies for the first time after surgery. In Vietnam, the parents' reaction was much different; they were so quiet, almost stunned, when they came into the recovery room and saw their children for the first time after surgery. They were more serious, but you could sense how much they cared, how precious their children are to them.

—*Betty*

RECOVERY ROOM NURSE
PORTOLA VALLEY, CALIFORNIA

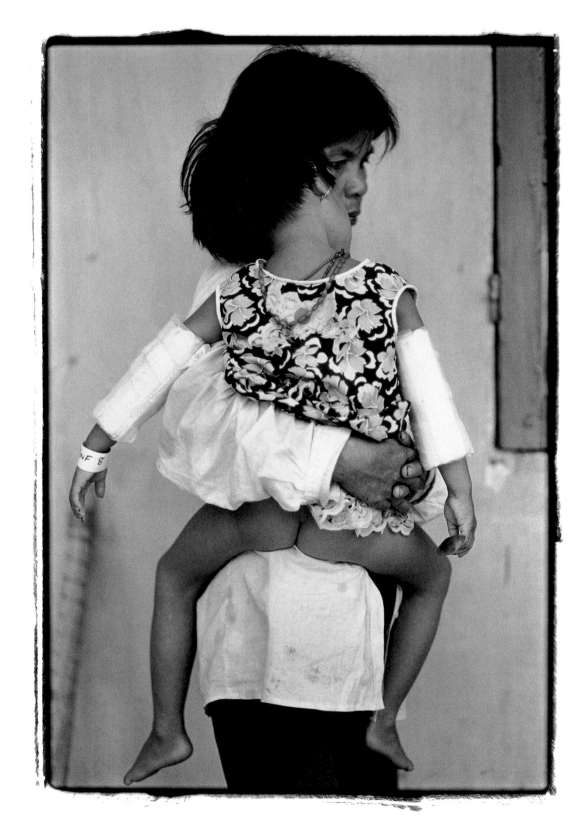

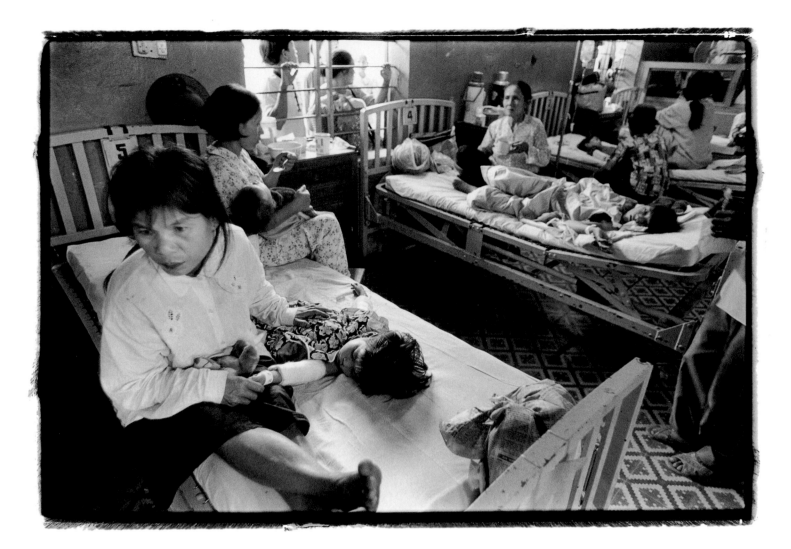

It really didn't surprise me that Hoi's mother didn't have a huge burst of emotion after the operation. I think partly she was dealing with a huge fear factor. First of all, she's living up in the mountains—to come down into the busy city, with the street activity and all that, that's got to be frightening. But then also dealing with these western people . . . as far as I know, she'd never seen a white man before. Then doing these strange surgeries and performing this "magic" on her kid . . . it would be akin to an alien coming in and reviving the dead or something! That degree of fear has something to do with it.

—*John*
ANESTHESIOLOGIST
DANVILLE, CALIFORNIA

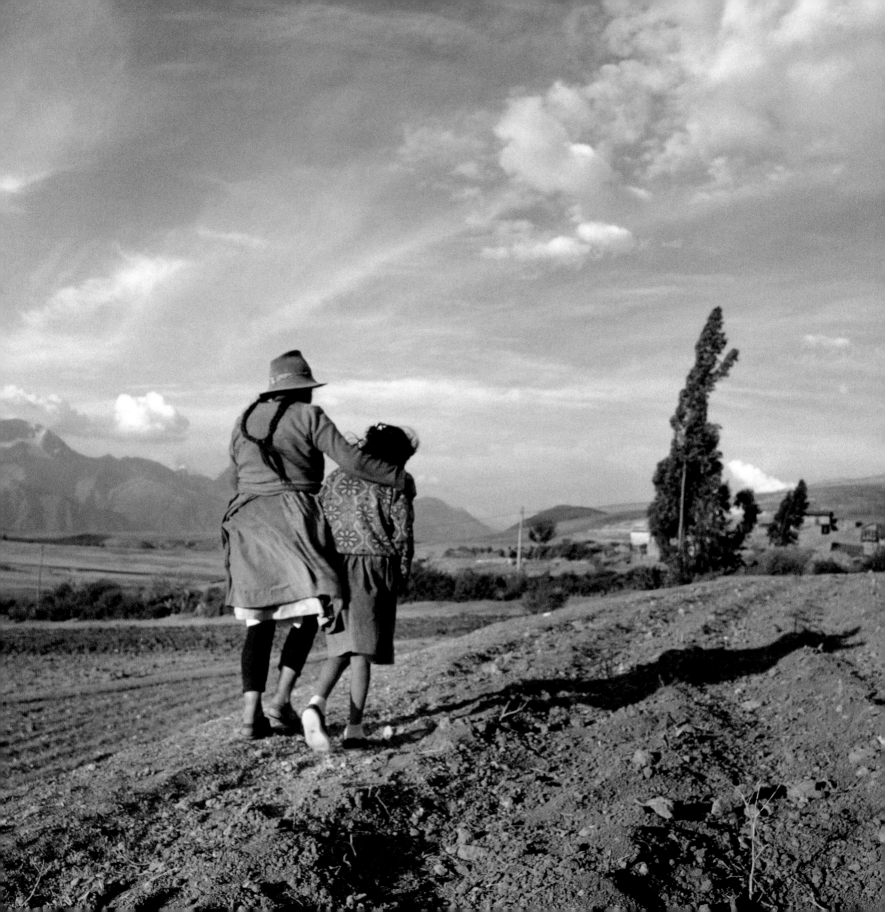

isabel

Isabel lives with her parents and six brothers and sisters in a
two-room adobe house in a village high in the Peruvian Andes. A neighbor listening
to his radio heard the government announcement that the Interplast team was coming.

He ran over to tell Isabel's father, Lucio. Isabel's family immediately made plans
for Lucio and Isabel to make the long journey to the hospital in Cuzco, in hopes that
the American team would be able to help.

The accident happened two years ago. Apparently, Isabel was playing or cooking outside when some kerosene ignited and set her clothes on fire. Cooking burns
are very common in countries like Peru, where kerosene is frequently in use.

Of all his six children, Lucio said, Isabel was the one blessed with beauty. She
was always a very happy girl and an excellent student. She still has two good friends
in her village who accept her as she is, but since the accident many of her classmates
seem to be afraid of her. She cries and runs away when they tease her. Lucio said,
"Ever since Isabel was burned the whole family is occupied with sadness."

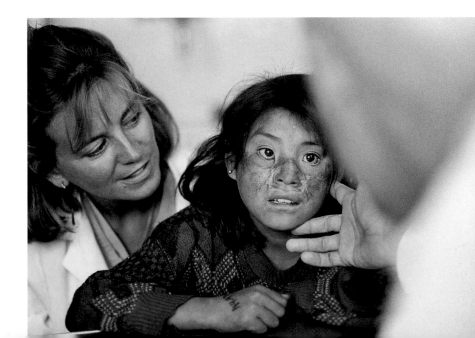

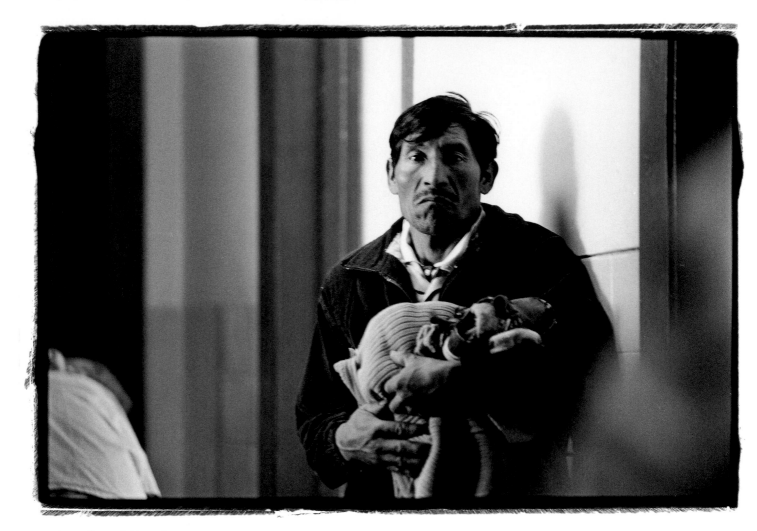

Lucio watching Isabel leave for surgery.

The children here are so stoic. They leave their parents and are taken away by strangers who don't look like them or speak their language. There was this little Quechua girl who got off her mother's lap, took my hand, walked right into the operating room, hopped up on the table, and helped us hold the mask to her face.

—Barbara
RECOVERY ROOM NURSE
SALT LAKE CITY, UTAH

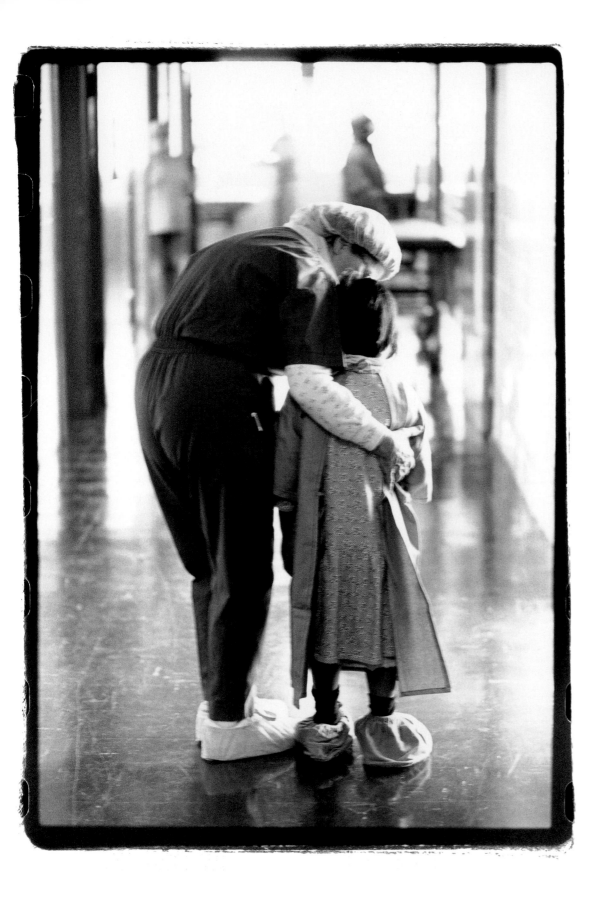

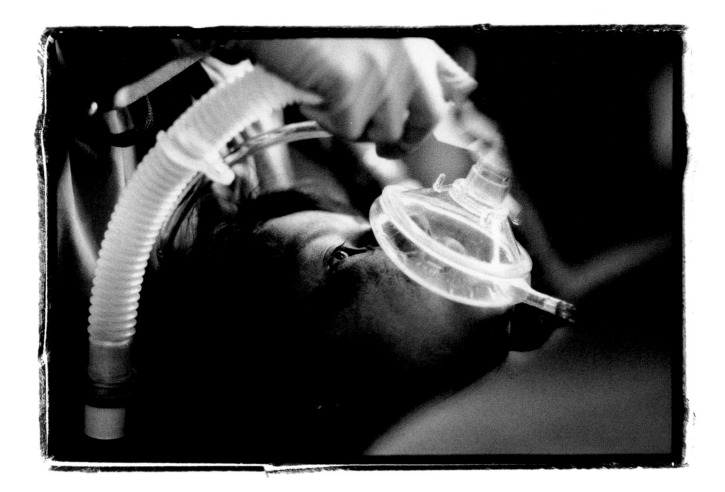

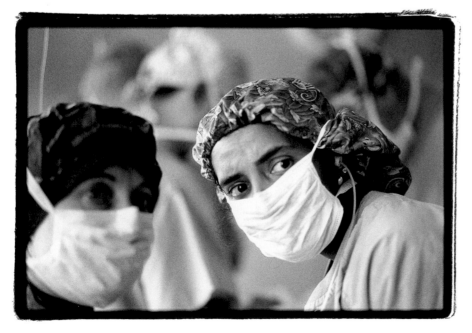

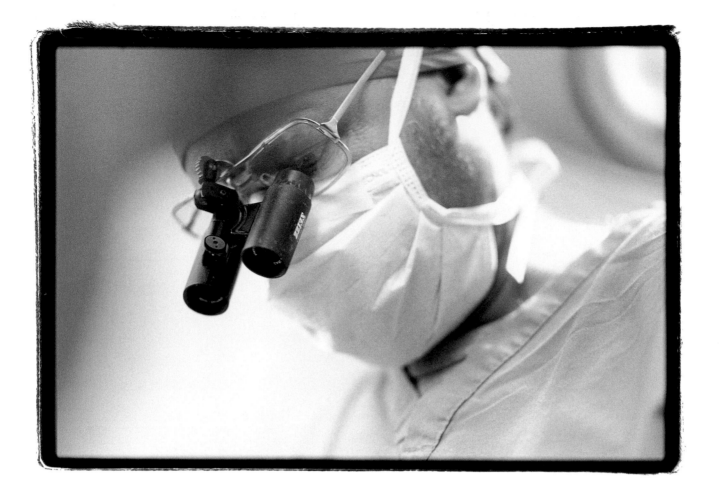

Facial burns are never easy. Our main objective was to release the scar contractions that were pulling Isabel's lower eyelids down. There are several treatment options in a case like this—it's a matter of weighing the options.

—*Tony*
PLASTIC SURGEON
ST. LOUIS, MISSOURI

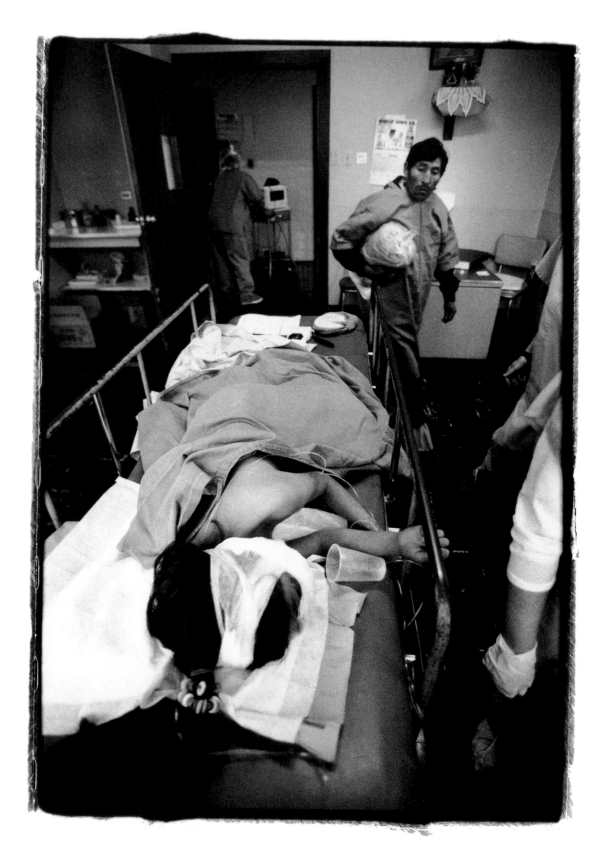

Lucio's first look in the recovery room.

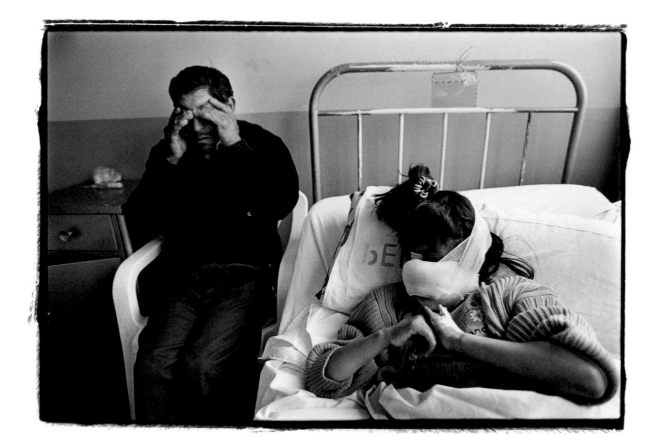

With her face heavily bandaged to help hold the grafts in place, Isabel spent the whole night being sick to her stomach. I remember her father, Lucio, spending the next three days in the ward, until she was well enough to be released. To sleep, he would curl up on the floor next to her bed.

—*Maureen*
RECOVERY ROOM NURSE
BERKELEY, CALIFORNIA

The operation took three hours, and it was three days before Isabel could go home. Two weeks later, I made my way up to her family's house in the mountains. Lucio was working in the potato field when I arrived. Isabel immediately ran off to get him while her mother and grandmother began preparing a large lunch of potatoes and eggs. I tried to peek under the bandages to see how the grafts were healing, but was afraid I would disturb them. Tony had told me that it would take six months to a year for the result to look its best.

—Phil Borges

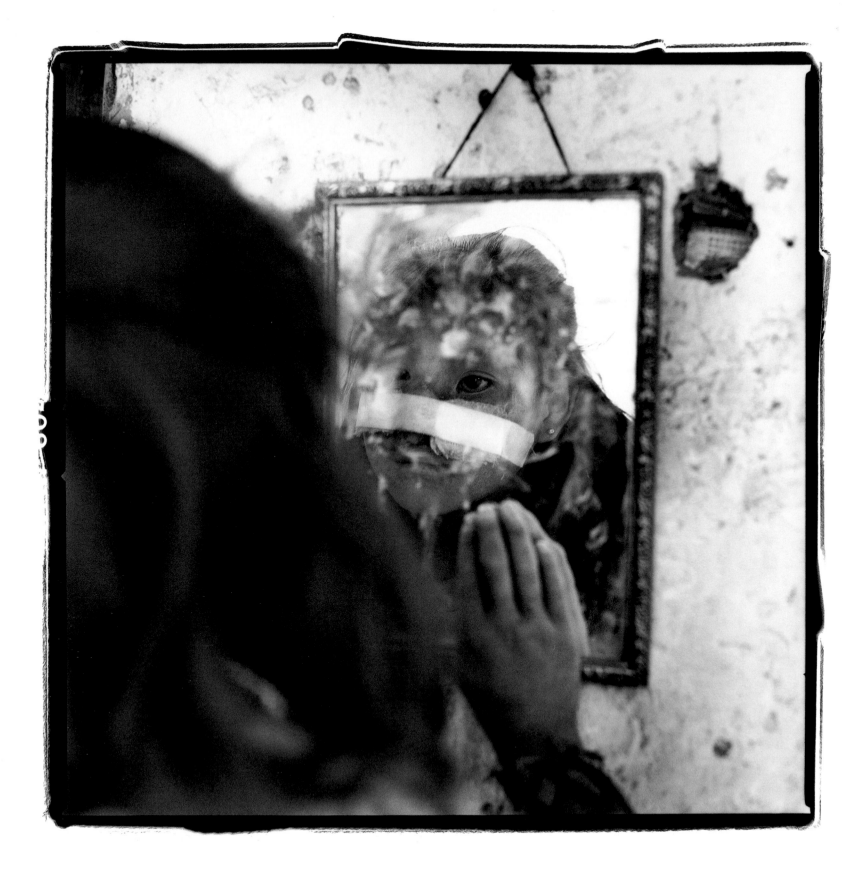

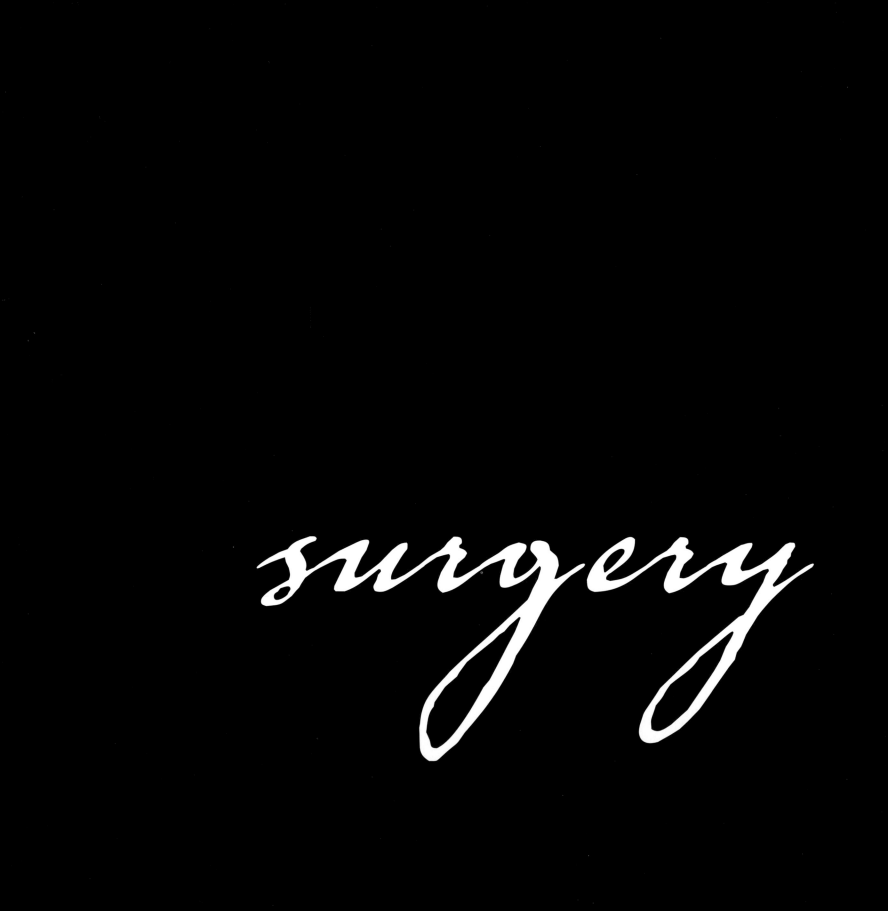

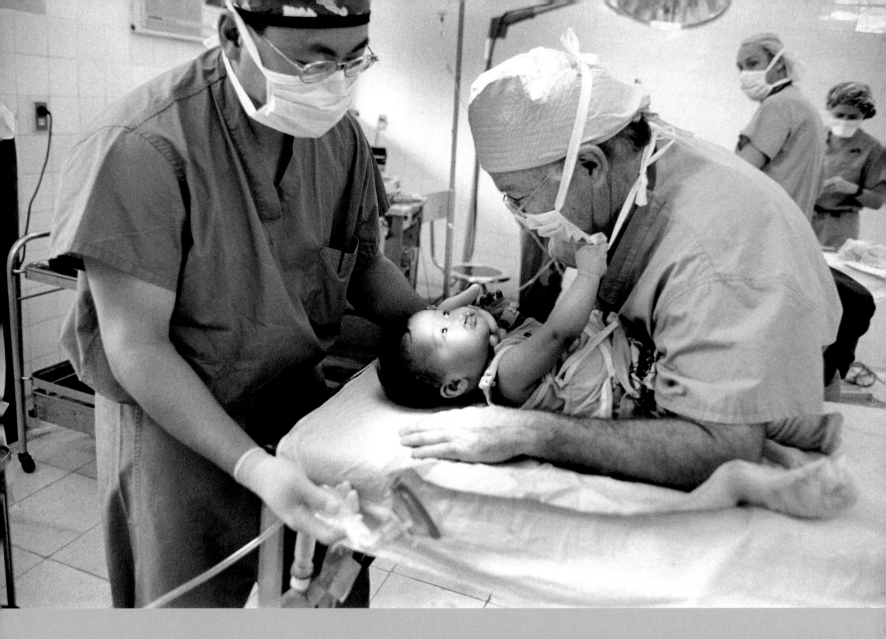

A CLEFT-PALATE OPERATION IS A RELATIVELY straightforward procedure, but cleft-palate surgeons operate in a sea of bacteria. Any mouth operation is considered a dirty operation; it's just the nature of the beast. Fortunately, given the typical Interplast operating-room environment, DNA has programmed into humans the defense mechanisms necessary to make mouth surgery possible under even relatively austere conditions.

An Interplast team's initial encounter with a typical operating room is often an eye-opener. Interplast teams can count on little beyond the basic shell of the room, the furniture, the sinks. There might be a gurney, an operating table, a fixed light, a sink, a suction machine, perhaps a rusty cylinder of oxygen in the corner. Little more. The buildings might be substantial, but the operating-room floors are often bare cement. In Peru, the windows were open; insects came and went. Mice were evident in Quang Ngai, along with an occasional cockroach in an equipment box.

Preparing for anesthesia, Hoi An.

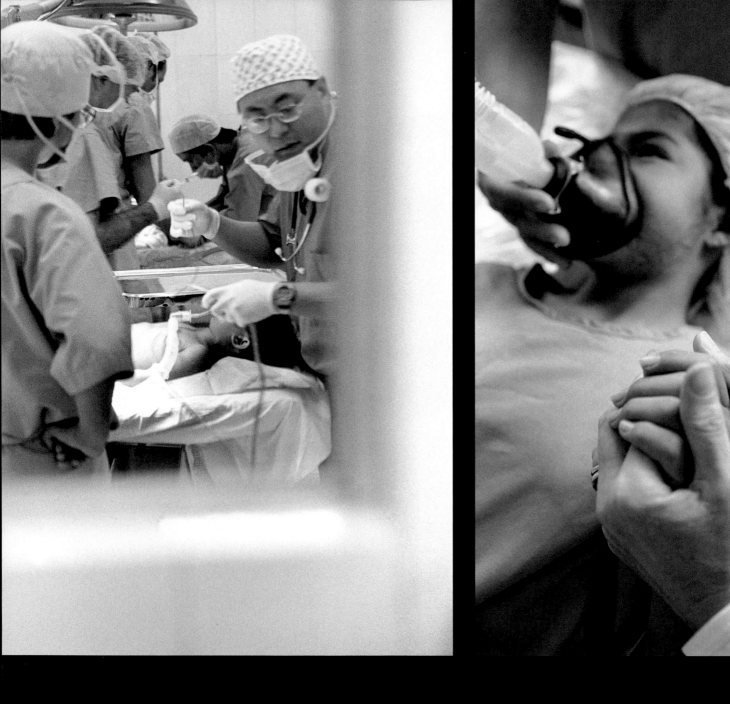

As the typical screening continues, however, the operating room transforms. Interplast sends all the necessary equipment—perhaps twenty large crates carrying half a ton of oximeters, autoclaves and other sterilization equipment, paper products, gauze, syringes, IV bags, medications—plus toys for the kids before surgery and clothes for them afterward.

In Peru, where the equipment arrived a week late, the team had to get started without supplies. The surgeons began performing minor procedures immediately using available supplies and local anesthetics.

Such conditions teach medical teams from developed nations eye-opening lessons about concepts like waste. In modern Western hospitals, the paper products alone from a single surgery will fill a garbage can. Once, after several days of surgery in Peru, an American nurse noticed a local nurse washing out her disposable surgery hat. *No, no,* the American thought, pointing to a large box of paper products, *just get a new one and throw it out after each operation.* Some time later, the American nurse learned that her counterpart had been lovingly cleaning and reusing the same hat since Interplast was there last, more than a year before.

Every available volunteer joins in from the very first preparations. It's something like a barn raising; hierarchy barely exists. The pattern of mutual support and assistance spills over into every aspect of the team's work. Immediately and dramatically, a group of strangers is far more integrated than they would be back home. The whole team is involved from the very beginning to the very end of each day, when they make rounds together.

In a Stateside operation, everybody is behind a mask; team members might not even know some of the people they're working with. And each, of course, has his or her own very prescribed duties. In a hospital in a developing country, the limited equipment and resources generate intimate scenes that suddenly seem

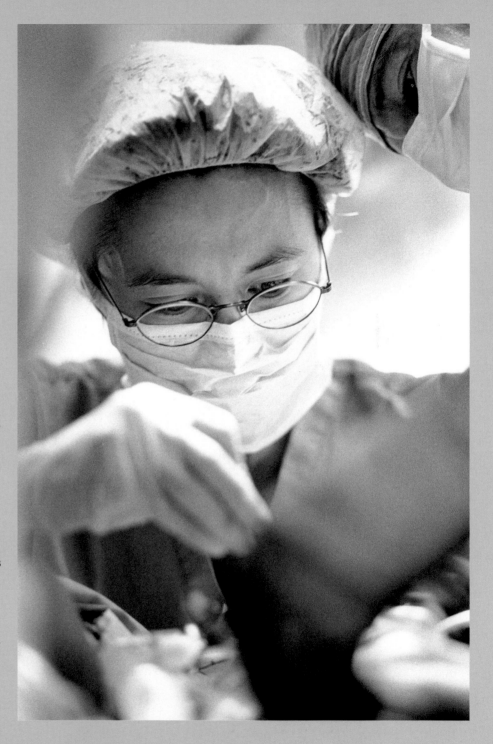

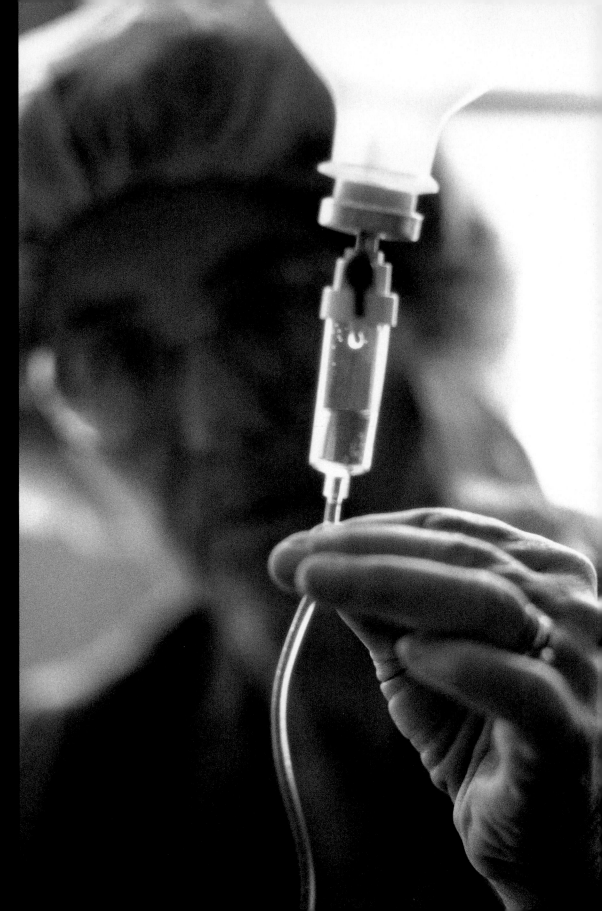

In Peru we screened 216 patients and completed 99 surgeries. And we essentially did two weeks of surgery in the last week, because all our supplies were delayed in customs. Going into the second week, we all knew how hard it would be. Such long days! We were doing surgery from 6:30 in the morning until 10 P.M.— then we would do rounds. All the time, new patients were still coming in to be screened. But everyone pulled together; even though some nurses could have gone to bed, they stayed up as late as the entire team— everyone really gave 150 percent. You really felt that we were all there to pitch in, to help one another out.

—*Dawn*
OPERATING ROOM HEAD NURSE
MORGANTOWN, WEST VIRGINIA

strangely missing from U.S. operating rooms—scenes like a post-op child being transported to the recovery room not on a gurney, but in his doctor's arms.

The speed and efficiency of the work, out of necessity, are also dramatically different. In Peru, as soon as the equipment arrived, two surgeons had two tables in use twelve to fourteen hours a day. In Vietnam, three tables were in use.

The sense of faith is plain during surgery. You can see it on the team members' faces. There's enough confidence—and hope—to get them through. But that hope is measured, and the outcome is never assured.

The sense of faith is even stronger for the patients. For them, it must be like encountering something from outer space. When these white-coated, masked strangers take your baby from you, you might have only a rough idea of what they can do—and you can't even talk to them. There are interpreters, yes, but it's not uncommon to communicate thirdhand through two interpreters—one who speaks English and Spanish, for instance, and one who speaks Spanish and the Quechua dialect of the patients in Cuzco. And yet the level of trust is astonishing.

Time and again, the medical teams rise to the occasion. Sometimes they must get by with as little sleep as they can manage without compromising safety. Sometimes they must improvise under unexpected conditions, as in Peru with the missing equipment. But even there, the atmosphere in the operating room is one of joy, not drudgery. People feel good working together as a team, they feel good about what they are doing—and they get constant, revitalizing feedback from patients, parents, and relatives.

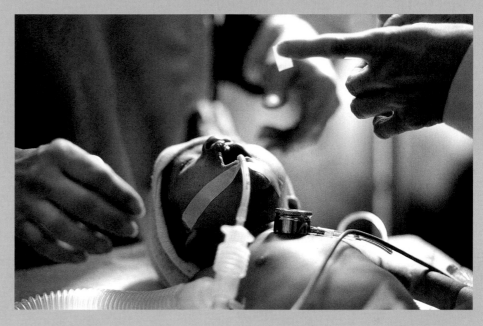

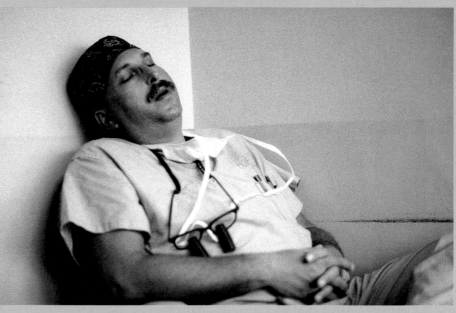

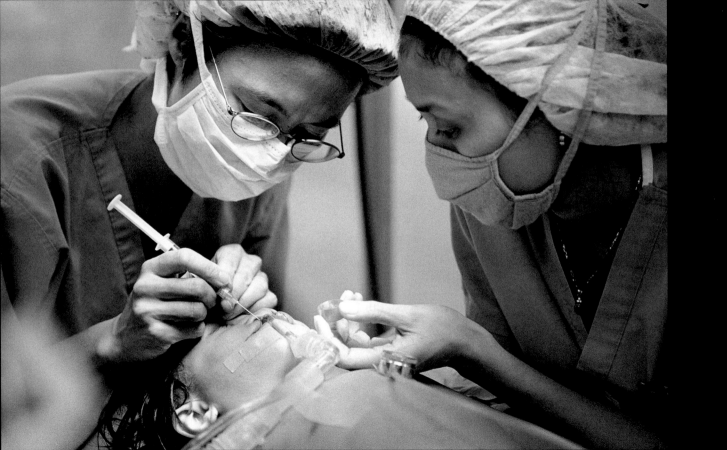

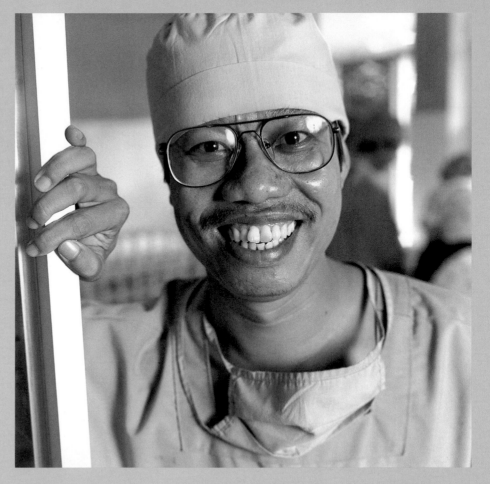

Dr. Tran Van Do was very inspirational to me. Here was a guy who survived the Vietnam War, though he wouldn't talk about any of the things that happened to his family. He got himself educated, and now he goes to great efforts to learn modern anesthesia. He has learned English as best he can, because English books are where he's going to get information. And then he teaches what he knows.

He worked so hard on this trip, to be sure that we were taken care of and to learn as much as he could. I mean, it drove some of us batty! Because he was just right behind us with one question or another, trying to get in on things. But I loved being with him, because he had such boundless enthusiasm.

I was blown away when he told me what he makes—something like $17 a month. He's obviously not doing it for the money, which is so much of what drives modern-day medicine in the West. This guy does it because that's what he loves to do. And he does it from a deeper sense of mission. For him to do anesthesia is a tough job, because he has so little to work with. I remember someone asked him, "Do you have everything you need? Are you happy with this?" And he said, "Oh yes—I have a moped, and I live in a nice little house with my family." And he was very content.

Then I came back to the States and had to deal with all these other physicians who whine and complain about the littlest things—and I do the same thing! But I just thought, "This is so petty—the things we complain about here are so small in comparison." It's a therapeutic perspective to get. For Dr. Do to say, "I make $17 a month and I'm content and happy"— that's an extremely different definition from what even the poorest in the United States would define as happiness!

—John
ANESTHESIOLOGIST
DANVILLE, CALIFORNIA

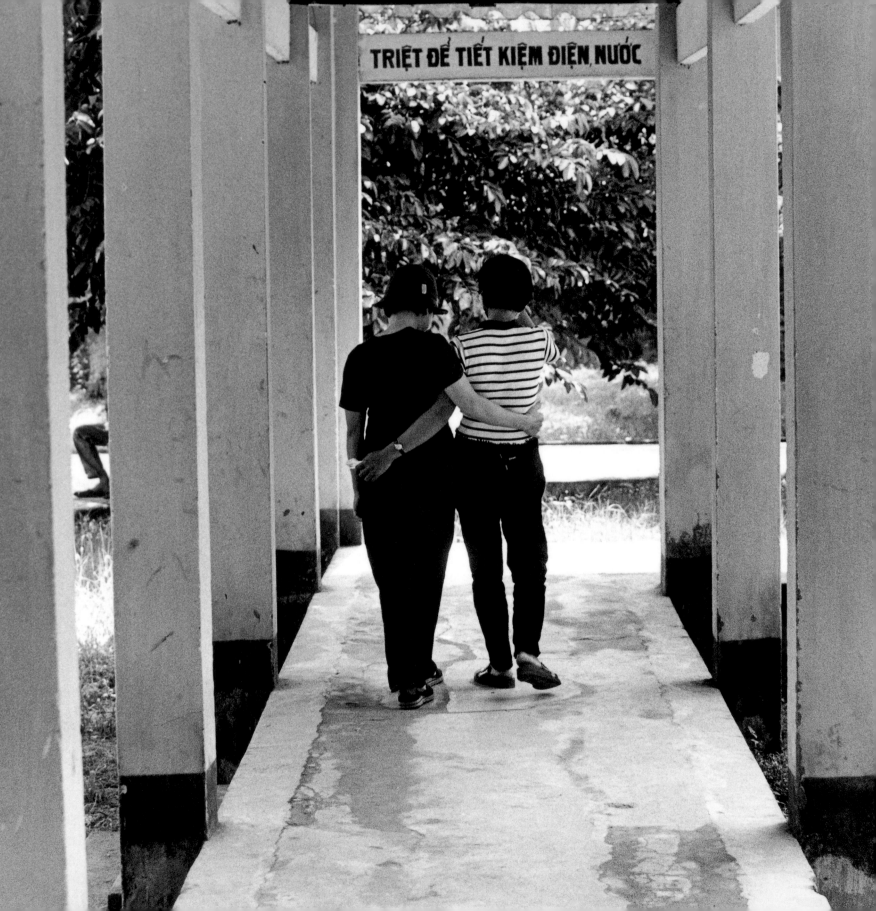

bay

Bay, who lives with her mother in a village of about thirty families near Da Nang, was a teenager when Interplast visited. Although her cleft lip was accepted in her village, Bay would never have thought of venturing out of her community without covering her mouth.

Bay, who has never gone to school, said she has no hopes of having a family. She has never had a boyfriend—but, more importantly, she said she would never want her children to live through what she has had to endure.

Lien, her lifelong friend, had heard about Interplast two days before the team arrived. She told us that she had always felt so sorry for Bay, and never thought that a cure would ever be possible for her friend. Lien could hardly believe it was true— the thought that Bay's deformity might actually be repaired.

At first, Bay didn't want to make the long trip to the hospital. She felt it would be useless. Lien kept encouraging her, and Bay finally consented. For five days Lien stayed by her friend's side, encouraging her throughout the entire process of trip, screening, operation, and recovery. Everyone on the Interplast team was impressed and moved by the strength of their friendship.

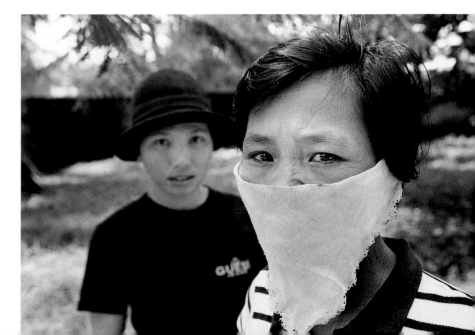

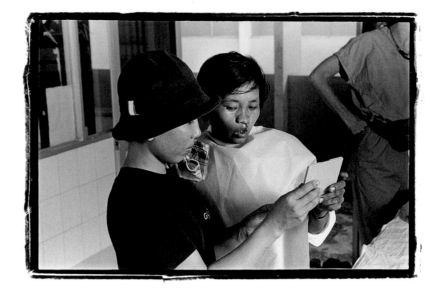

Bay was afraid, because she didn't know what surgery was, and she wasn't sure how it was going to turn out. From what she understood, surgery was like cutting something from the body, and she was afraid. But her friend talked her into talking with us—she was using her handkerchief, and she wouldn't take it down. Her friend was trying to tell her, "It's OK," trying to comfort her, you know, because everyone here looks the same, other children have the same deformities—and finally she kind of took it down. But even after the surgery, she was still using the handkerchief to cover her face, and she didn't want to use the mirror.

She was so embarrassed, yet she had so many hopes of what she wanted to do in life, that only because of her deformity she was unable to do. She wanted to join society, do something good, learn about things, but she couldn't do it. It was just kind of like a dream for her; she wanted to fulfill her dream, because she couldn't really work, other than just in the rice field, and stay around the village.

Bay really touched me. Her best friend took such good care of her. They were not even related and the friend, Lien, was much older . . . I think twenty-four.

They were born in the same village. Lien went to school, but Bay did not because of her deformity. When Lien heard about Interplast she got all excited. And I'll never forget what Lien told me after the operation was complete. She said, "Oh, Bay looks so much better. You know, she is really beautiful. . . ."

—*Jennifer*
INTERPRETER / SECRETARY
NORTHRIDGE, CALIFORNIA

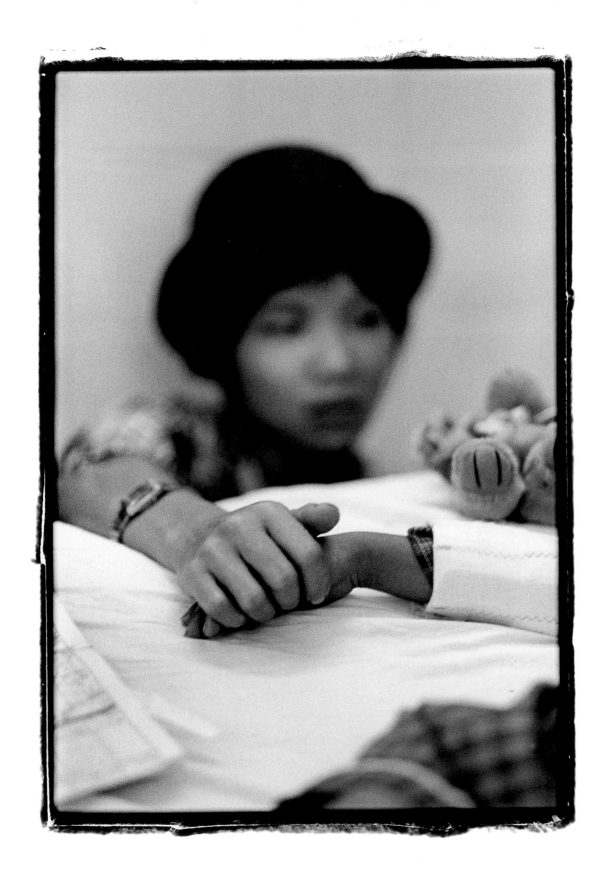

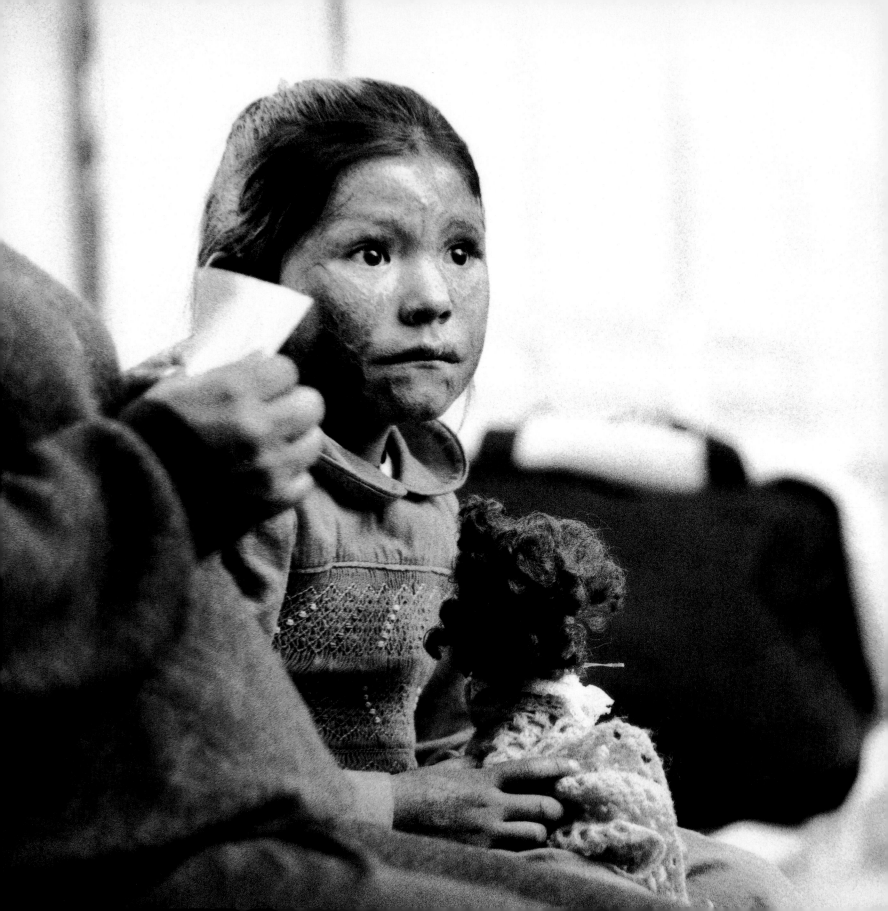

ester

Ester's father left her mother when Ester was just two years old.
Her mother began drinking more frequently and was intoxicated when a cookstove blew up and severely burned Ester's face. Two months later, Ester was taken to an orphanage in Cuzco.

Julia, a nurse at the orphanage, has taken Ester under her wing. She told us how Ester loves to sing, dance, and write poems. When Julia heard the announcement on her radio that Interplast was coming, she could hardly wait to tell Ester. On the day of the screening, Ester put on her favorite dress, grabbed her dolls Margherita and Angelina, and walked with Julia to the hospital.

Unfortunately, there is no easy treatment to correct the damage done by a burn. In Ester's case, Paul, the surgeon, decided that the most that could be done was to release some of the scar contractures on her hands and face to give her greater mobility.

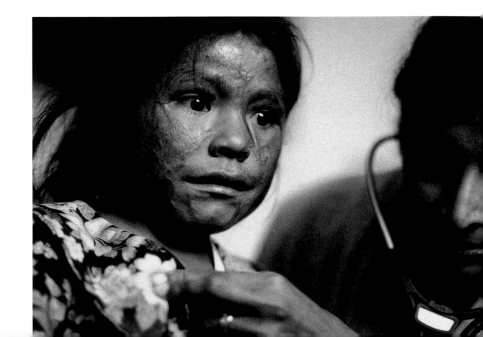

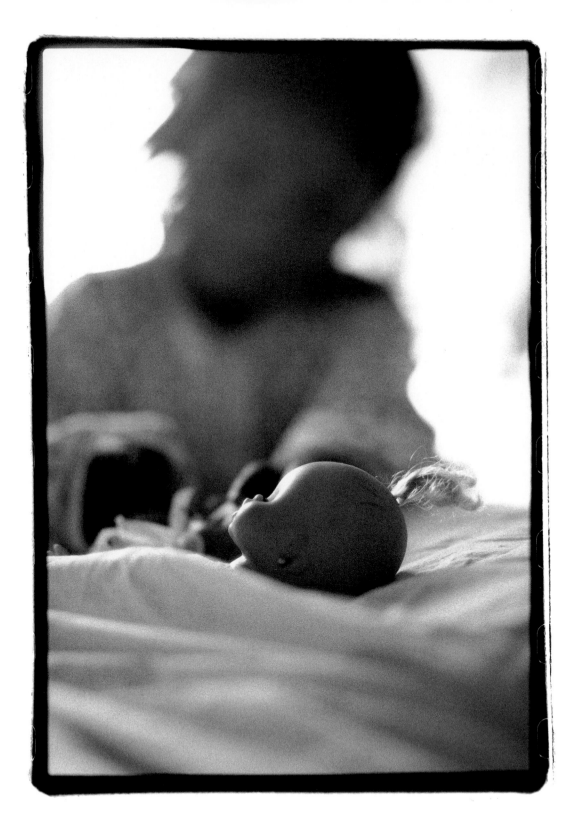

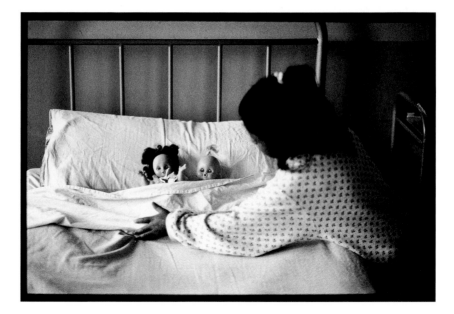

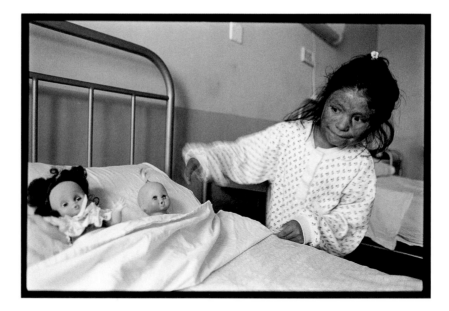

*We came by on evening rounds and here was Ester, tucking her dolls
into a spare bed, assuring them that the next day would be all right.
This seven-year-old orphan, entirely alone on the eve of her surgery,
attending to her loved ones . . . it really moved me.*

—*Elaine*
PEDIATRICIAN
ALBUQUERQUE, NEW MEXICO

Compared to working at home, you're a lot looser here; you feel a lot more freedom to voice your opinion or to say exactly what's going on. At home, you tend to be more formal; there are a lot of hospitals where you don't call the physicians by their first names. But on Interplast trips, titles almost seem to drop. We're not so caught up in titles; everybody's there to do the same job, and however we can get that job done, then that's how it gets done.

—*Abby*

OPERATING ROOM NURSE
SALT LAKE CITY, UTAH

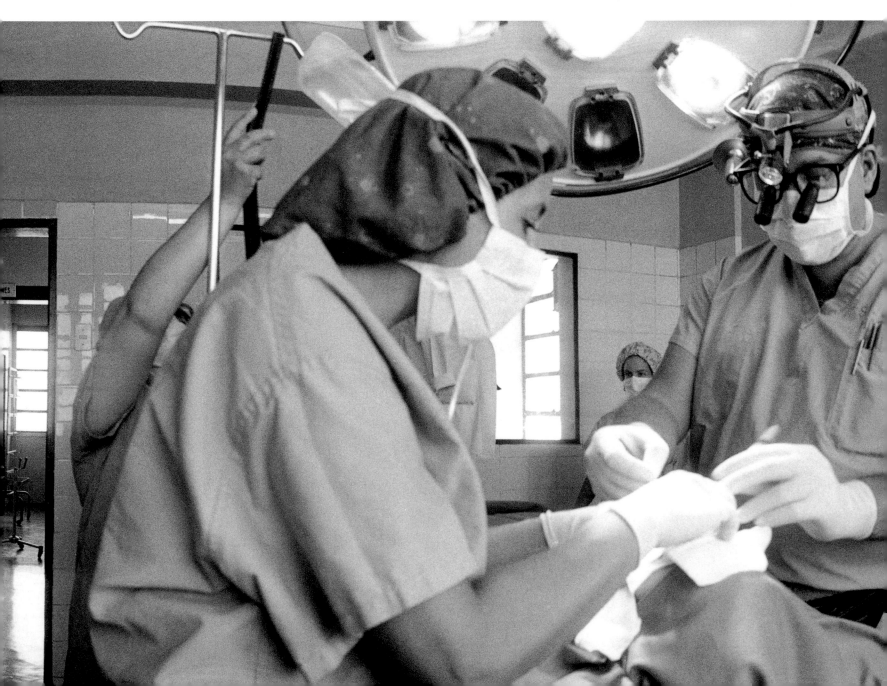

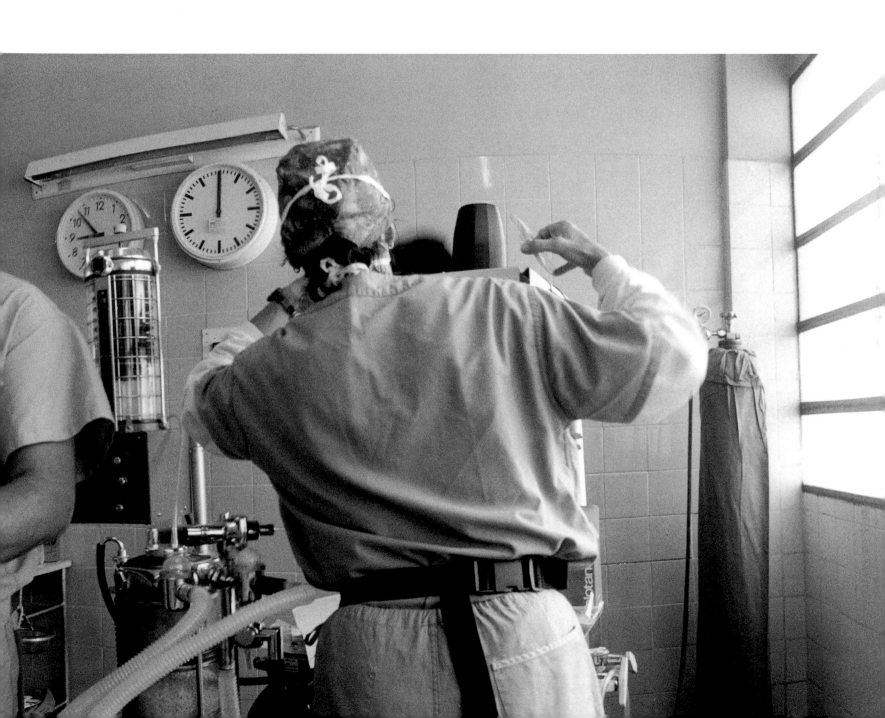

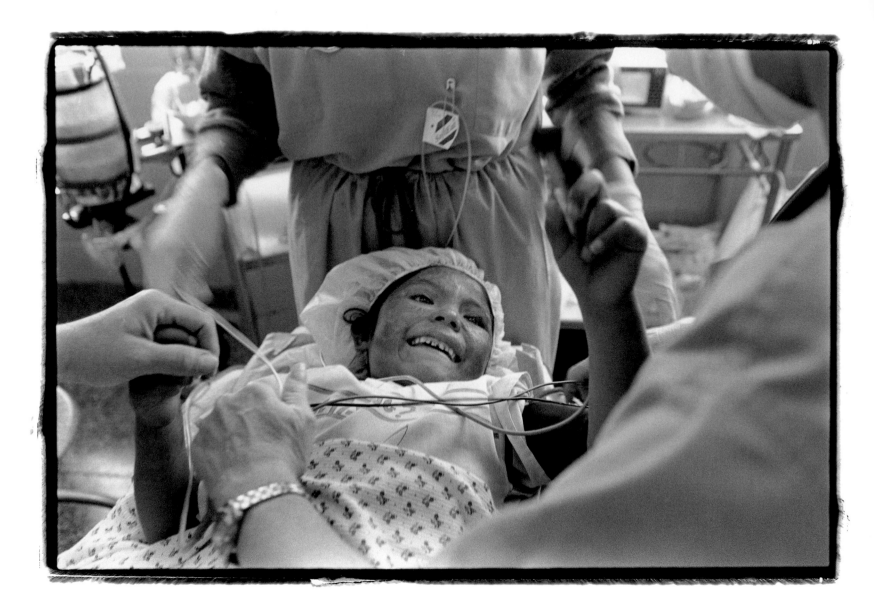

Julia told me that Ester went back into her shell at the orphanage—always withdrawn. But when she visited Julia's house, three nights a week, she opened up and came to life: singing, dancing, writing poetry. Here she's moments from going under anesthesia, but she's cheerful and lively. She loves attention!

—Phil Borges

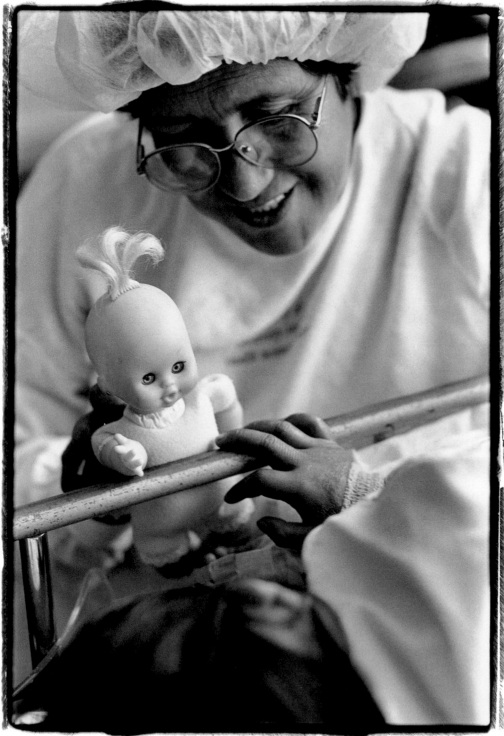

Julia and Margherita greeting
Ester following her surgery.

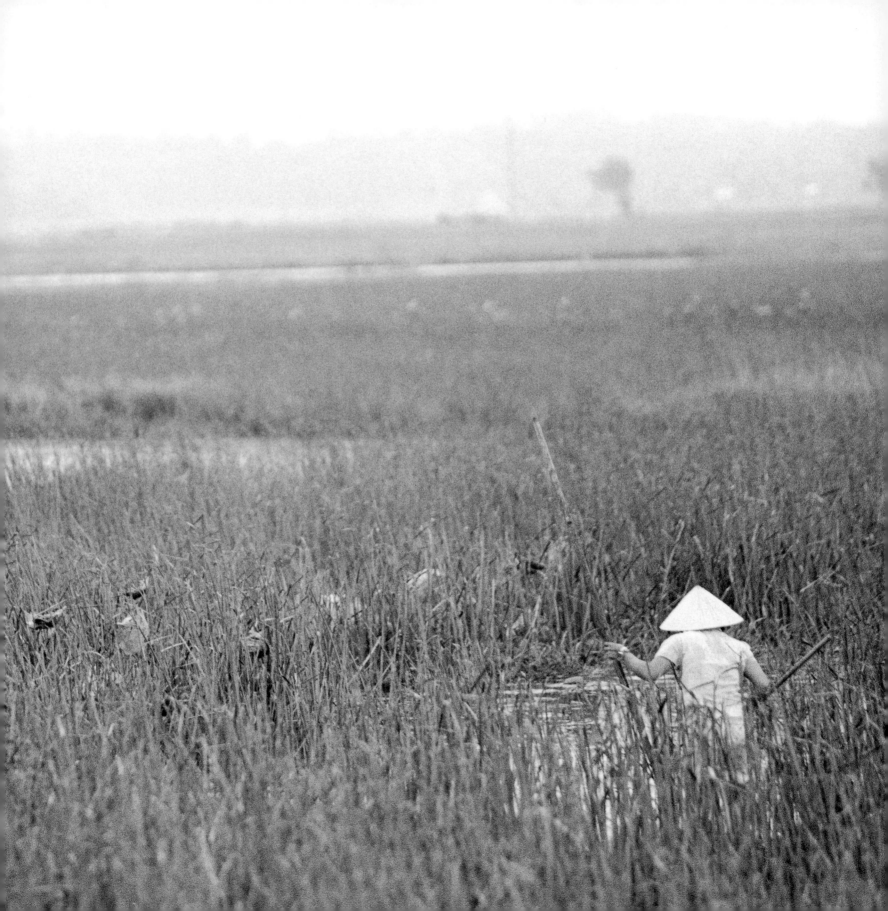

Lan

Lan, the youngest of six children, lives alone with her sixty-
four-year-old mother, Doithi. Their tiny village, Tinh Chau, is just two kilometers
from My Lai, site of the Vietnam War's most infamous massacre. Doithi vividly
remembers hearing the shooting and seeing the fires burning the houses. Terrified,
she ran and hid with her children. Lan was born three years later.

In Vietnam, there is a prevailing belief that if a pregnant mother sees a child
with a cleft lip, her own baby can "catch" the deformity. Children like Lan are therefore typically isolated.

Lan has been extremely shy all her life, and spends most of her time working
alone in the rice fields. She is Doithi's only child to not go to school; she has never
had a boyfriend or even a close girlfriend.

Lan was twenty-two when Interplast visited. A month or so before the team's
arrival, Doithi came home from the field to find her neighbor waiting to report
about the coming American surgical group. Doithi recalled, "I was so happy I
couldn't stop crying all night."

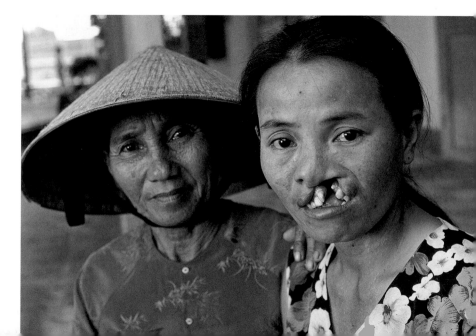

When I first learned I was going to Vietnam with Interplast, I wondered whether we would be met with some residual hostility from the war—especially since the hospital we were going to was close to My Lai. But the people were so warm and gracious—not just the patients, but strangers I met on the street. It was amazing.

—*Alice*

PEDIATRICIAN

BERKELEY, CALIFORNIA

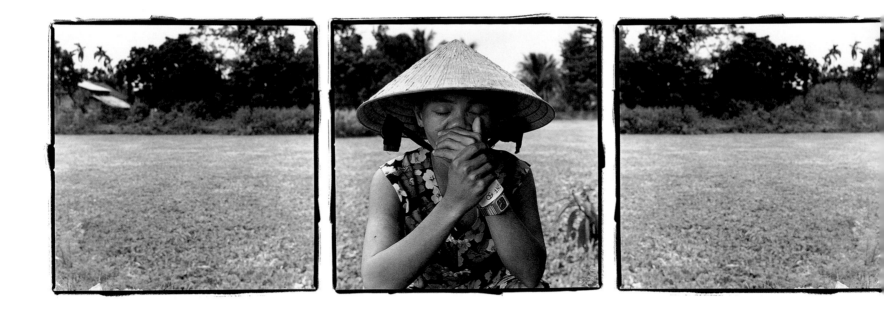

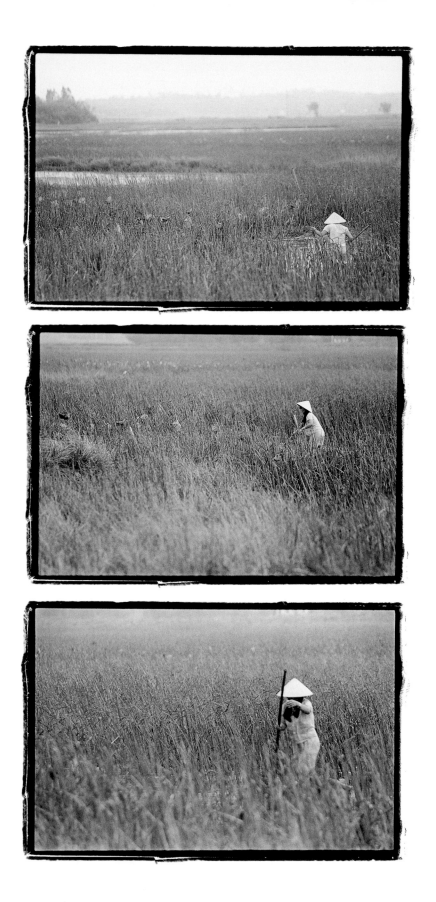

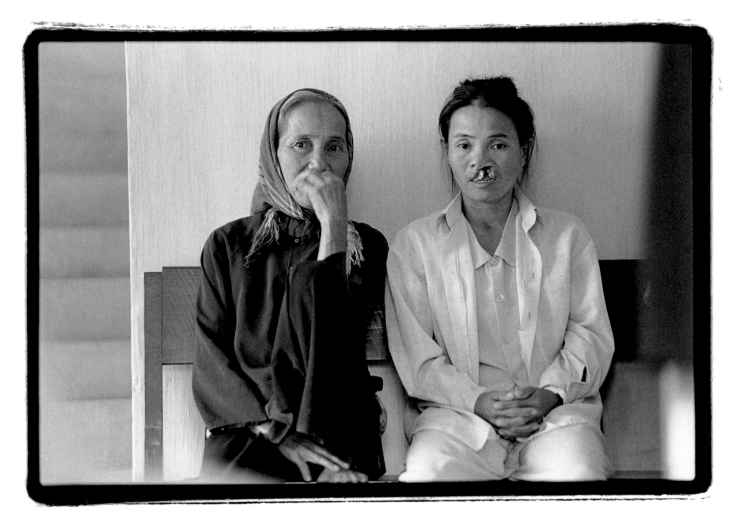

It can be pretty shocking when you first see an
adult like Lan with a cleft lip . . . but what
struck me most was the fact that she was such
a beautiful young woman. It's thrilling to be
able to do something very minimal that can
make such a huge difference in someone's life.
                                              —Gary
                                    PLASTIC SURGEON
                        MARTHA'S VINEYARD, MASSACHUSETTS

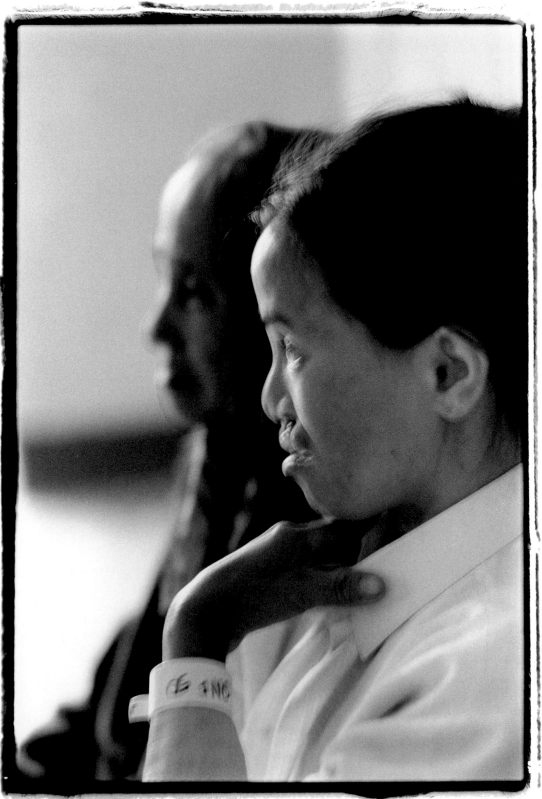

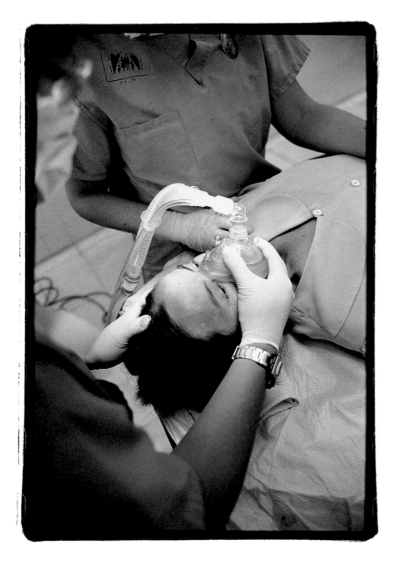

Opposite: *Lan's neighbor anxiously awaiting the out-come of the surgery.*

The operation took a little less than two hours. Gary, the surgeon, spent much of that time trying to reshape the cartilage in Lan's nose. After twenty-two years, the nasal cartilage was so rigid and had such a strong "memory" that, ideally, a second surgery would be performed later to continue reshaping her nose.

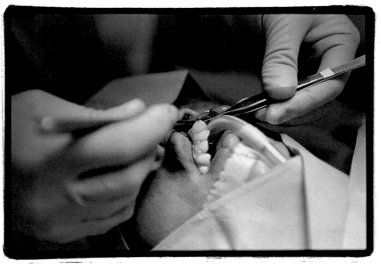

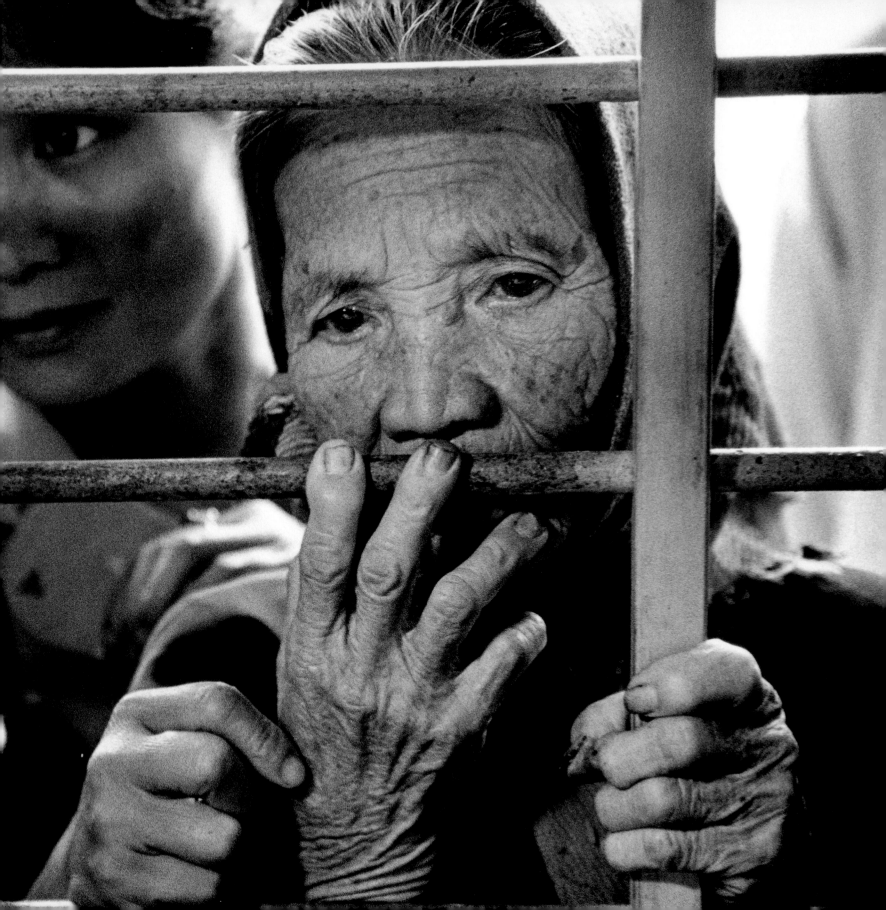

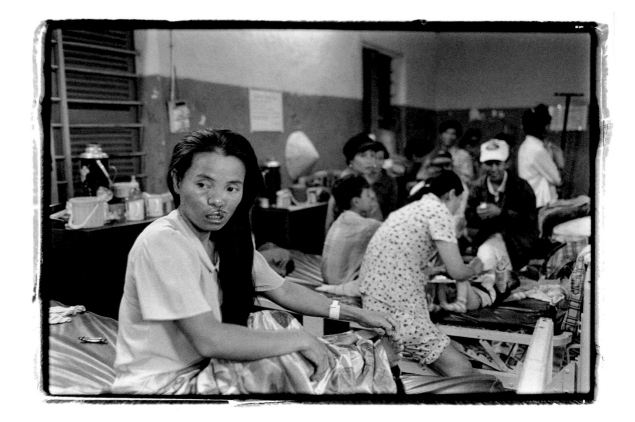

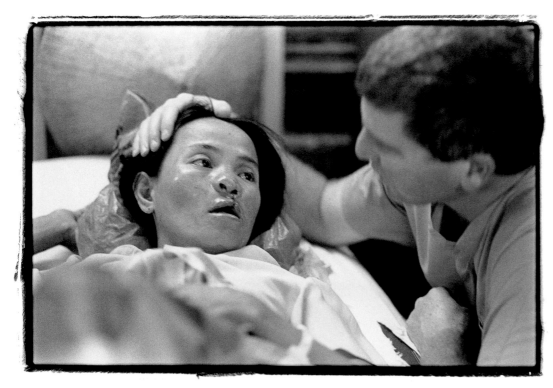

During the whole procedure, Doithi and their neighbor anxiously waited outside the recovery room. When the surgeon first gave Lan a mirror after the operation, she just looked and stared for the longest time. Doithi had stared in the same way before Lan fully regained consciousness. It seemed to be a look of mingled fascination and disbelief. In a way, they were looking at a stranger.

It wasn't until the next day that Doithi told us how happy they were.

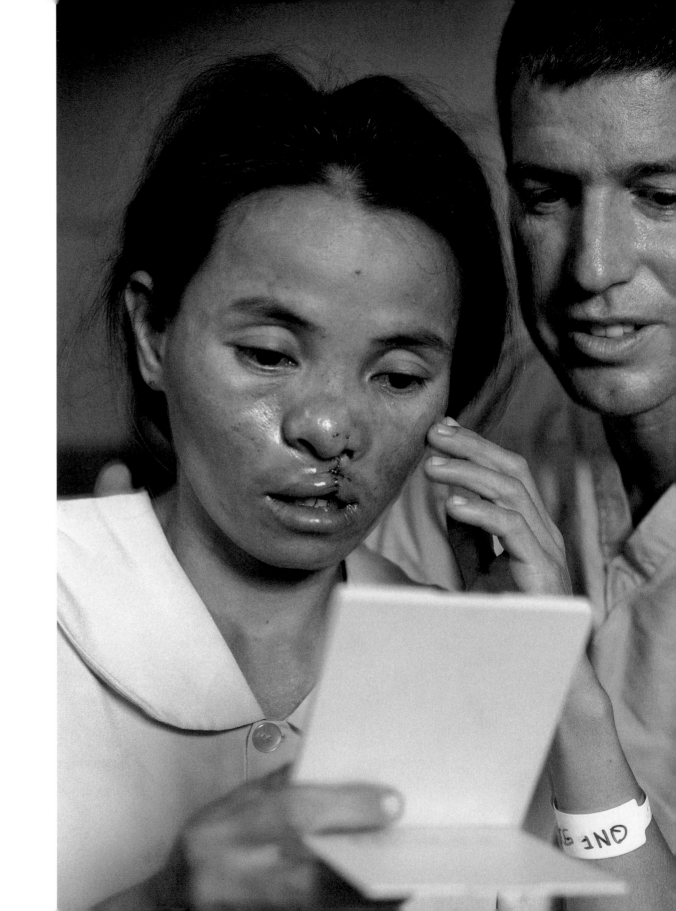

Lan, four hours after surgery.

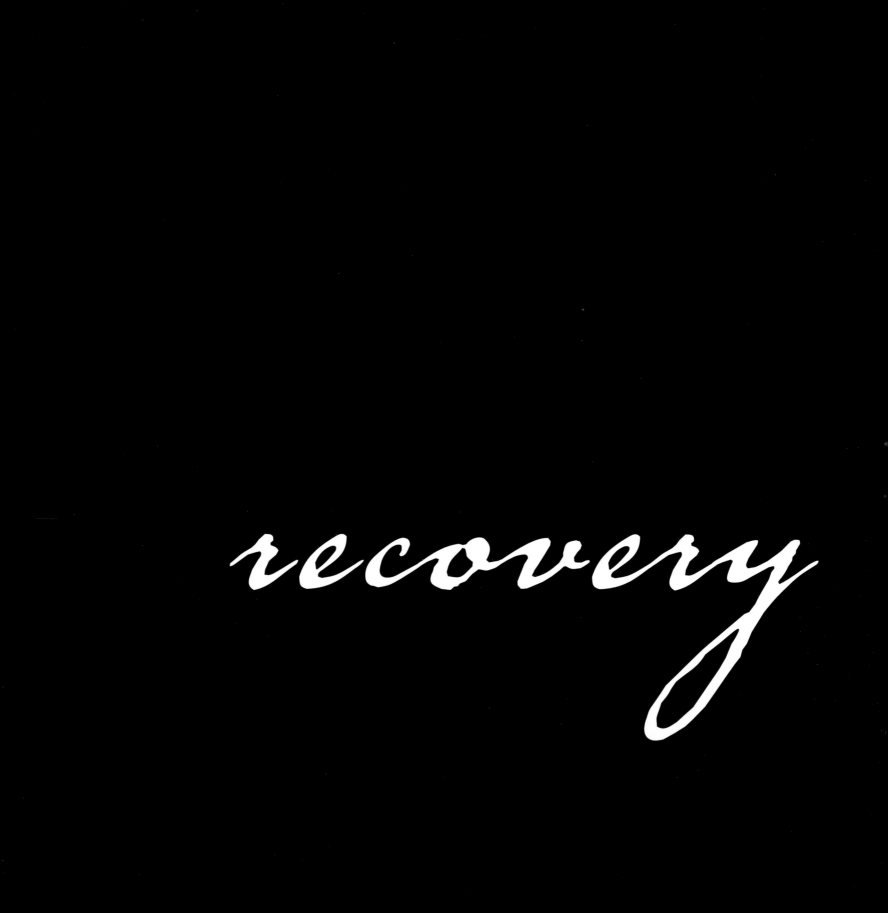

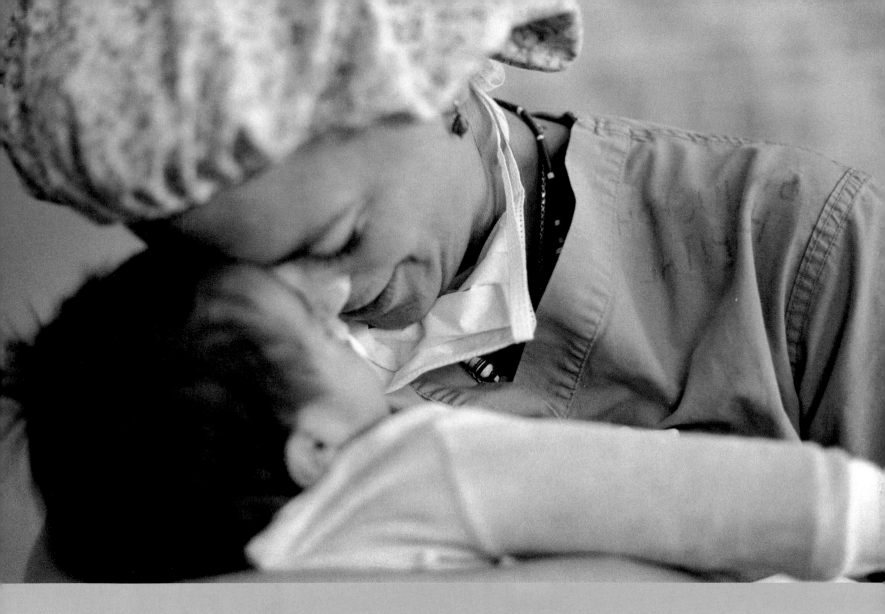

IMAGINE THE FEELING OF JUST WAITING WHILE your child or grandchild or family member has been taken away and is being worked on by strangers who don't speak your language. Waiting. Waiting for your baby to come into the recovery room. Perhaps you have come from your home far out in the country. You may never have been in a hospital before.

The families have to trust that the team knows what it's doing—they have to have the confidence to get them to that hospital—just as any of us have to have faith when our children go to a doctor in a developed country. But here it is a step removed, because the doctors are from a different culture. After all, it's just hearsay that the Interplast team is good at what they do. The local people don't know how good; they're taking a leap of faith, and they just want to see their children get better. The patient is gone for only an hour, an hour and a half, sometimes a little longer in the complicated cases. But that waiting period, that anticipation, is always moving.

In the developed world, parents are not generally allowed to join their children in the recovery room.

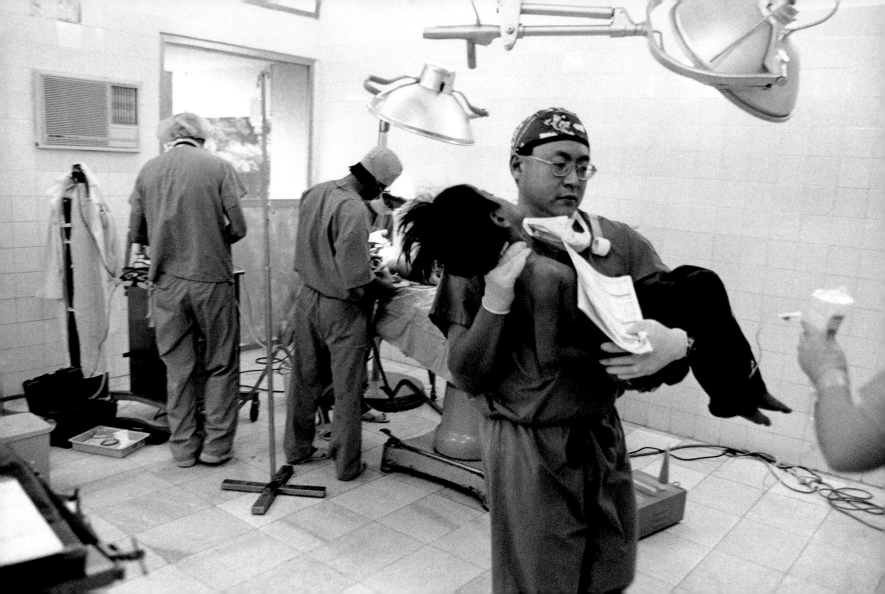

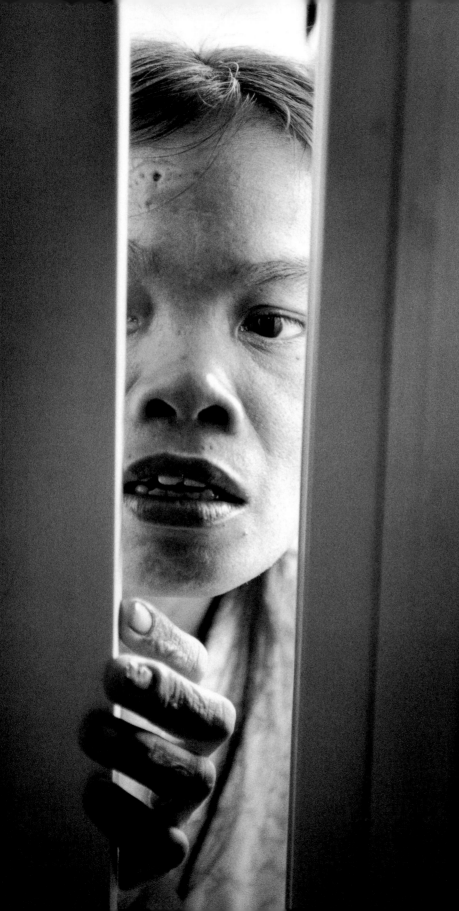

Mother waiting for her son at
recovery room door, Hoi An.

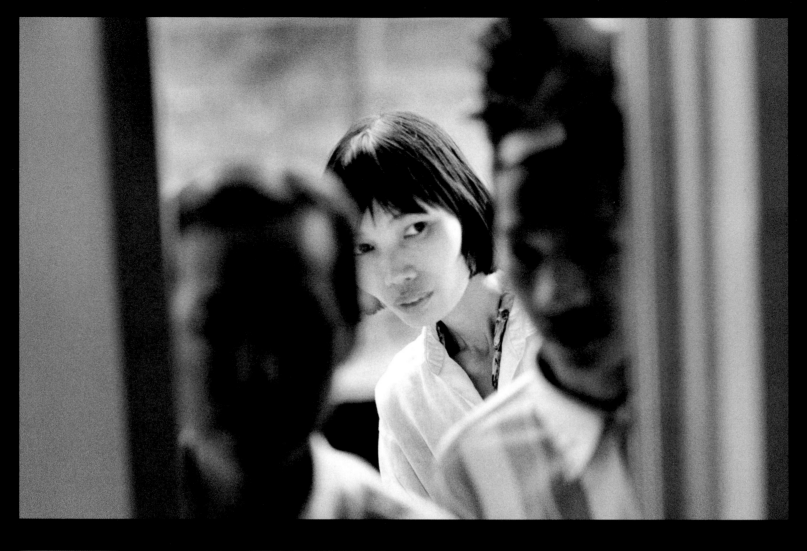
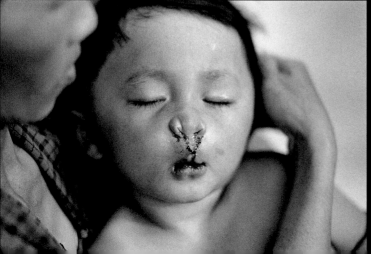
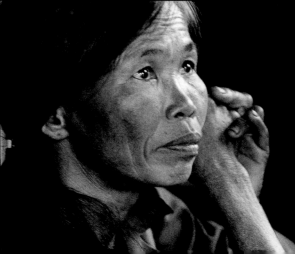

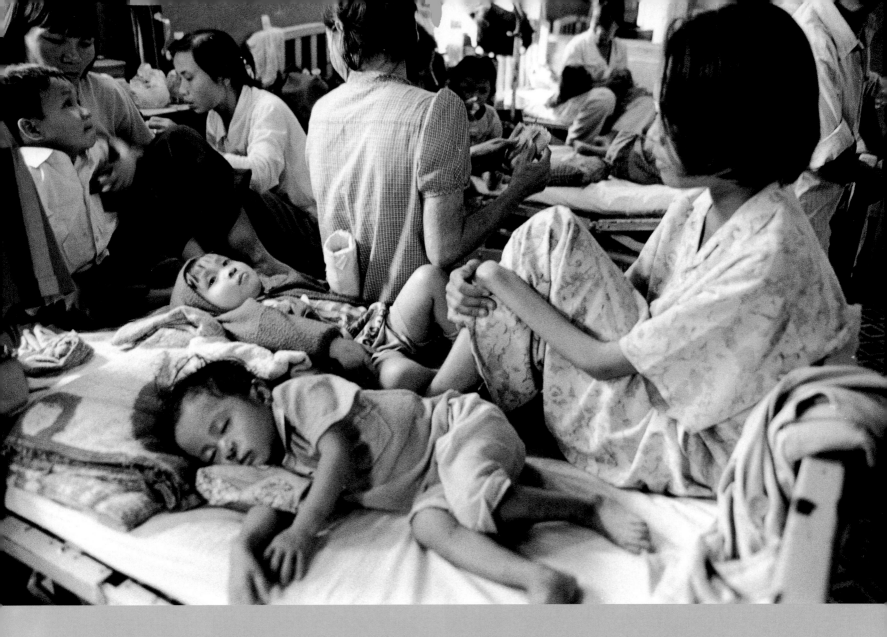

But Interplast nurses often gown the parents and bring them in immediately after surgery, to ease the apprehension of both the child and the family.

A recovery room or ward in a Western hospital would never have a dozen beds, with four to six babies per bed, each lying horizontally. The families of each of those patients crowd around, with more people outside the windows, waiting. It would be impossible to get everybody supporting the patients into the room. At times, family and other supporters literally surround the building, remaining for an entire week, twenty-four hours a day.

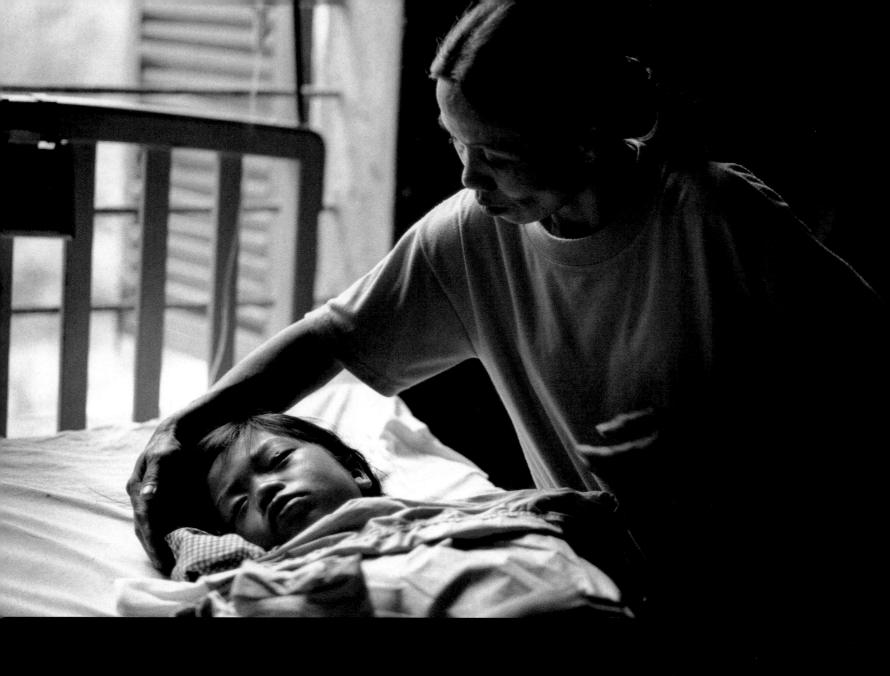

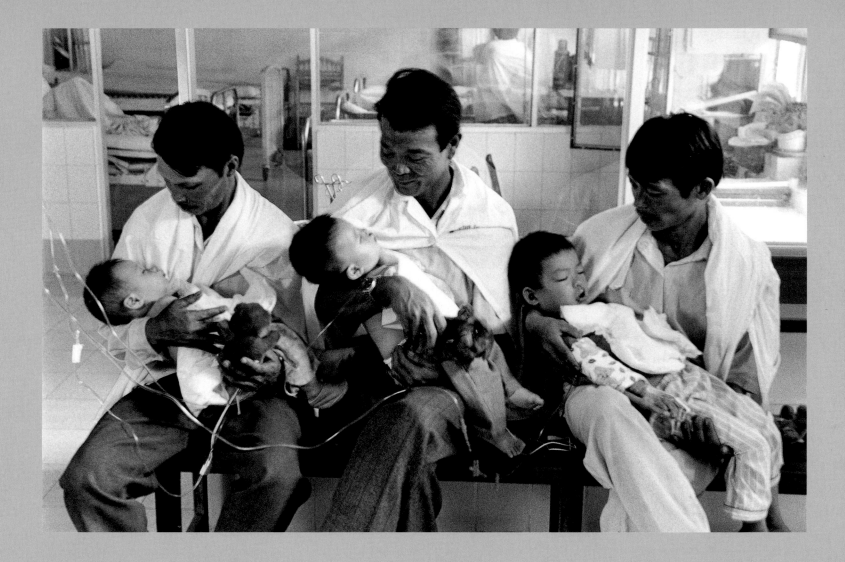

The fathers in Vietnam were always there, always involved. They were sent by the mothers into the recovery rooms first, because it was too emotional for the mothers to see their babies right away.
　　　　　　　　　　　　　　　　　　　　—Phil Borges

terri

I've said to people

who've never been on a trip and are nervous about it: "You're going into the army, but it's the spiritual army, and you volunteered to be there." What I mean by that is that it's kind of like a MASH unit; you're going to have a good time, and your spirit is going to feel so good, and that's why you're doing it—because it's a spiritual experience. It has nothing to do with money.

ANESTHESIOLOGIST
PALO ALTO, CALIFORNIA

I went into medicine because I wanted to take care of people, I wanted to make a contribution. But often that can get lost. Most of us can get caught up in trying to achieve, trying to be the best, worrying about medical or legal things, earning a living . . . and so as far as taking care of people and being compassionate—it starts to recede as a priority. On these trips all those extraneous reasons are removed—no one is making money, becoming famous, exerting control in the hospital, or finishing up quickly to get home to the family. When I go on trips like this, caring becomes the number one reason—and that's so pleasing to me. I am just there to give what I have to give. It's very pure, very freeing. I come back feeling more at peace with myself.

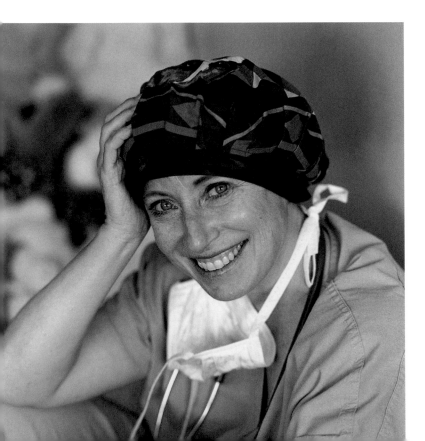

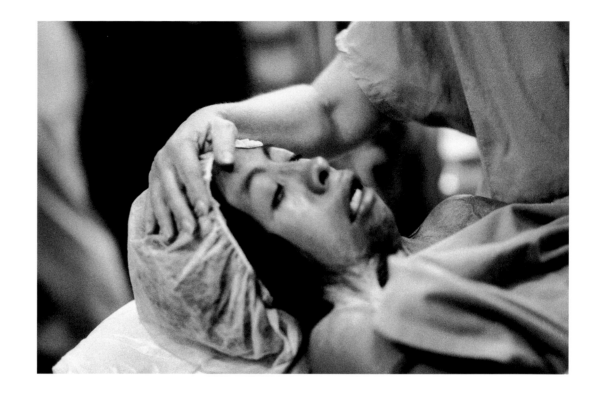

This may sound insincere, but I don't mean it that way: I think I owe this. I have a skill that is so easy to transport and so useful, and I've been making a good living for a long time, and I'm in good health. It seems incredibly selfish of me not to share it.

I don't think that anyone who is fortunate enough to live well should get away with not doing volunteer work. This is what I've chosen. It's fun, and gratifying, and I get a lot out of it: learning about other cultures, going to places I wouldn't otherwise visit, learning how to function medically in an environment that is not at all ideal, learning how to be flexible, how to be creative, how I can make things work when I don't have the ideal equipment. That's translated into my practice; it's made me better at what I do. It's an adventure; and it also allows me to relax a little bit and work hard—and by "relax" I mean that I can take my time, I don't have to look at my schedule, I can talk to my colleagues and get to see the patients afterward.

john

South America was a very different experience from what I got in Vietnam.

ANESTHESIOLOGIST
DANVILLE, CALIFORNIA

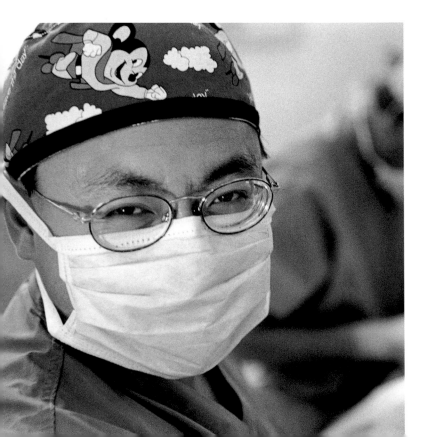

It had to do with the fact that I'm Asian myself, I think. It had a different impact on me in a way, seeing people of the same ethnic background as me. It hit home a little bit more, to watch the Asian parents with their Asian kids.

What I saw in them is what I would see in my own parents. I don't know how to put it into words, really, it's just a feeling. The interrelationship between the child and parent is very different in the Asian cultures. In Vietnam it was very much like the interactions I had with my first-generation Asian parents. The overall feelings are all the same, the parent wanting to protect the child and things like that. But a lot less is spoken; the emotions are there, but unspoken. And I can connect into that because I grew up with that.

The emotions were much more expressed in South America—you would see the moms cry when they saw their kids, or a father just beside himself with joy. In Vietnam I didn't see that, although I knew it was there, because my parents were the same way. My dad doesn't show his emotions, but you know they're right under the surface. *If you watch carefully, you can feel it. Watching the Vietnamese fathers be stoic reminded me of my father.*

You know, the things you have to deal with. . . . I still remember Abby had hooked up one of these suction machines—we were using one of the Vietnamese suction machines because ours was broken—and she turned it on, and it was whining away, making all this racket, in the back corner of the OR. I happened to look over, and the thing is smoking and sparking and all this stuff, and Abby just looks at me and puts her hands up in the air and shakes her head. . . .

That eye connection between me and Abby spoke volumes: "Here I am, so far from home, I'm doing these operations with this crazy equipment that's going to explode on me . . . but it's great!"

It's funny: the people on your team might be total strangers, and you'll leave, and you won't see them for two years or something; but you know that you'll come across them somewhere, and that connectedness will still be there. It doesn't go away. The experience is so stressful, but so challenging and exciting—and you share it with other people. It builds a bond that lasts.

I come back from these trips feeling inspired and rejuvenated by having witnessed the human spirit at work, having witnessed people who have a healthy spirit and know how to use it well. They don't look to the material world to find their solutions. They don't have the material world to look toward, they only have themselves and what their feelings and emotions are,

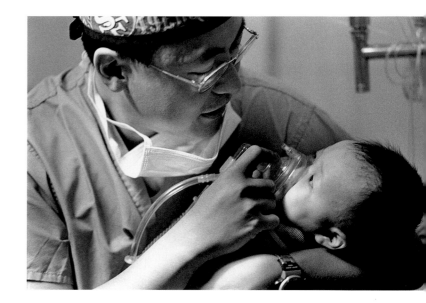

and their own inner strength. You can't help but feel touched by that. It puts you in tune with your own human spirit, your own sense of well-being.

Despair is an issue of the spiritual world, and that's where the solution is found—in the spirit, not in the material world. That's where you find the strength to deal with hardships. And I think that's something that is terribly degraded in Western civilization, because we're so caught up in the material. We think the solution lies in the material, and it doesn't.

For me, this realization created a bridge to be able to access that part of me more easily. Watching others deal with hardship helped me in my own way. And so, in that sense, I come back feeling stronger also—more at peace, more balanced.

brad

One thing that surprised

me was that we had quite an entourage, both with us and greeting us. Anywhere we went, we arrived and left in groups. There were always large groups of people there when you arrived, all the people waiting to come in, standing and waving, and holding their kids up. It made quite an impression, all these people waiting for you, when you realize they're all there because of you. You almost felt like a traveling rock star.

ANESTHESIOLOGIST
OGDEN, UTAH

It makes you feel like you're appreciated, and wanted, and certainly makes you feel that you're doing something worthwhile—especially hearing the stories about what some of the people had to do to get there, and how a lot of them really had nowhere to stay when they did get there—what they were going through to get their kids taken care of.

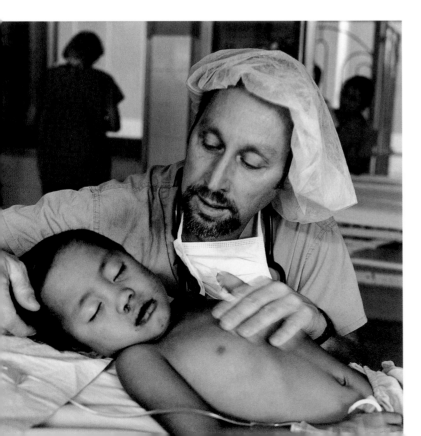

At home, you do the work every day and you take it for granted, and the people you work with take it for granted. That's probably the biggest change in medicine: we've gotten so good at it. Patients take it for granted that everything is going to turn out right, and if it doesn't turn out right, well then you must have

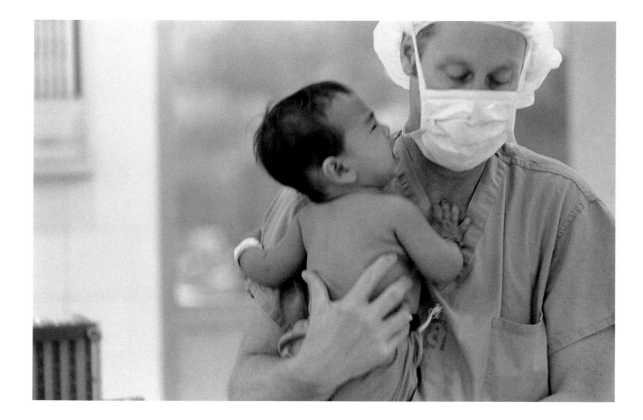

screwed up, we're going to sue you. It's actually pretty amazing stuff that we do every day, and it may become routine because we are doing it every day, but you go somewhere else where some of those things aren't available, and you realize what we really have at home.

This was clearly a team approach; everybody was pitching in, trying to get things accomplished, rather than waiting to do their special jobs. You get some of that in the OR back home, but it's more difficult because there are stricter rules. We had nurses running between cases,

so frequently I'd hand a suture or something to the surgeon, which is usually the nurse's job.

We didn't have the strictness of record-keeping. Half our record-keeping at home is for billing purposes, and half of what remains is for legal reasons. It was like a huge weight being lifted; all we had to do was keep records to document the care we gave, and we had the freedom to concentrate on just the procedure at hand.

abby

A lot of nurses who

OPERATING ROOM NURSE
SALT LAKE CITY, UTAH

go on Interplast trips save their vacation hours so they'll get paid for the time that they're gone, but even those nurses who don't get anything for their time away will say, "It's all worth it." Really putting your skills to use, and being appreciated, and feeling like you've done something that has made a difference, makes it all worth it.

No matter where you go, even though people may not be related, they help each other out. If mothers need to have their children at the hospital at a certain time, the news spreads like wildfire. Even strangers become like family. They help you get through what you need to get through to get your child better. That's what's great when you look out at all those faces, knowing they've all heard by word of mouth what they need to know. It's the same in every poor country I've been to—strangers all coming together at the hospital to help each other out, or before we even get there, passing on the information that we're on the way.

I think this work has changed me—well, in so many ways. One particular way is that now I try, even if it's just for a short time, to reach a patient I think I can

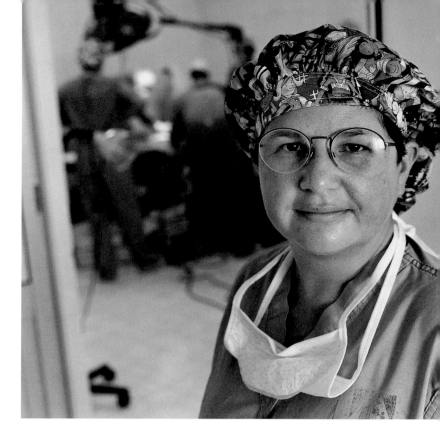

reach. The time that we have them in the OR—from the time the anesthesiologist says he's ready to put the patient to sleep till they actually do it—that's maybe only five minutes. I like to see if I can maybe help that patient feel OK in that little window of time.

I think before I went on Interplast trips, I looked at all the other things I could be doing in that space of time. Now, instead of worrying about charting, or counting sponges, I try to focus right on that patient, even if it is just for five or ten minutes.

In the States, we don't have the follow-up, the team camaraderie you have on an Interplast trip. Being so technical, and so made to look like you're just some-body going through the motions at the hospital, doesn't make me feel like I am anything other than a warm

body. When I go on an Interplast trip, I'm a lot more than a warm body, and everybody, including my own team members, makes me feel that way. Not just the families, but the people that I work with.

Nursing over the last several years has become so technical, so mechanical, that I don't think families realize all that nurses do. You go on an Interplast trip, and it doesn't matter whether you're a surgeon or a nurse or a photographer—they know that you're there to help, all of you together. You're there as a whole team.

And we get to see them afterwards, we get to find out how they are doing. The families then get a chance to say thank you.

In the States, you don't find anybody who says to you, "Thank you for making my kid's life better." Once in a while you do, but not very often.

jennifer

This was my first time

INTERPRETER/SECRETARY
NORTHRIDGE, CALIFORNIA

back to my country [Vietnam] since I fled in 1978 as a seventeen-year-old. I was one of the boat people, along with my mother and my two sisters. We had to pay twenty grams of gold each to get a place on the boat. I didn't fully realize the danger, but I remember being very frightened. We were being chased, and I remember the women dipping their clothes in the water and placing them on the engine to keep it cool. It took four days and three nights to get to Thailand. We had very little food and water. Dad had to stay behind.

Coming back is very strange. I hardly recognize Saigon. Such mixed feelings. I went back to our old house—everyone had changed so much. The neighbors all had grey hair.

We all have so much in the United States, but being back I can really see the difference. The parents in Vietnam are willing to sacrifice just about everything for their children. There was this one mother whose baby could not have surgery because he had a cold. She asked if any of us could take the baby back with us to the

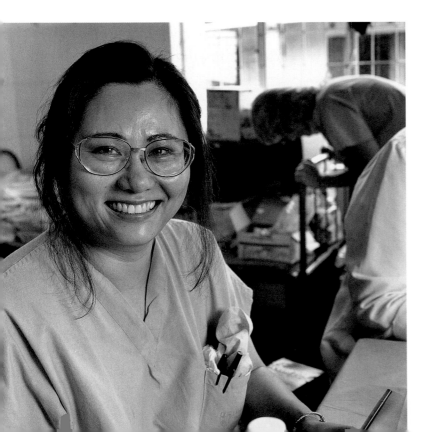

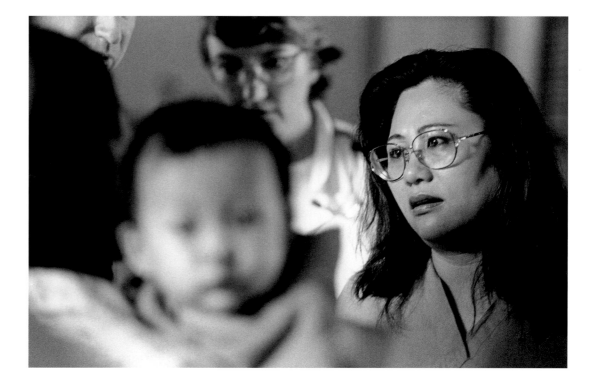

States to get help. At one point she told me she could give all the money she had to anyone in our group who could take the baby to the U.S. All mothers everywhere love their children, but this just amazed me.

I remember there was one woman who just froze on the spot—I guess, the shock—when her baby was turned away because he had respiratory problems. She just sat there in shock; we didn't see any reaction. I explained to her, but I don't know if she really understood. It just poked a hole in my heart.

Many of the parents who brought their children to the hospital were waiting outside for days, many times with little or nothing to eat. I took over some leftover bread and bananas and gave it to them. I can't get my mind off the trip. It really affected me. It made me feel like

I'm a very lucky person to have such a good life now. I realize how much better off I am than many other people. Now I want to share what I have somehow.

I wasn't in any medical occupation; I couldn't really do very much, so when I got back I wanted to go back to school and at least get something like a nursing degree—right now I am looking at joining the physician's assistant program. Hopefully, then I can do something. And even in this country (the States) I would like to do some volunteer work as well. This trip . . . it gives me more courage, because I saw the unlucky side of people's lives, and see that I am luckier, and I want to share that with other people. If I need something, I can afford it for myself, but these people, they can't help themselves.

Tony

It's wonderful to travel somewhere and get to do something while there, to actually get involved with the people. And to do fascinating, great surgery, where you have even more of a bonus—the immediate gratification of seeing a child, or even an adult, transformed before your eyes. It's such an intimate experience, being able to do that kind of surgery—on anyone, for anyone—but especially in a foreign country where access to such surgery is limited.

PLASTIC SURGEON
ST. LOUIS, MISSOURI

The group dynamic is interesting. It's hyper-real—an adventure on so many different planes, and you have to make it work. You're with the medical people a lot more than you would be in the States. You're traveling with them, living with them, socializing with them, eating with them. There's more cross-interaction between the surgeons, the nurses, the anesthesiologists, the support people, the other hospital staff. It's more congenial in many ways. There's not so much structure to put you in your proper places. That's a great thing you see sometimes. People's roles change from what they might normally be. Surgeons learn a lot about anesthesia, anesthesiologists learn about surgery.

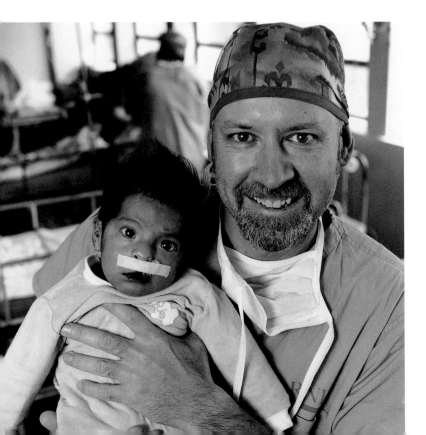

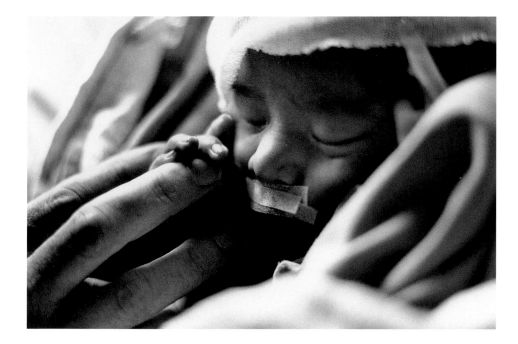

I've learned a lot on these trips. I've been able to do a lot surgically in a short amount of time, and that has really helped me. That's an obvious, concrete thing. I find I've been more tolerant of situations where everything doesn't work exactly right. I'm more willing to accept situations that might be considered a little more marginal, if the spirit is right.

The thing about Interplast is: you have to go for it. You can't have a can't-do attitude about it, because at every turn there's some looming disaster that's going to prevent you from doing it. And then the little things become so much less important: if your instrument is wrong, or if you don't have the exact retractor that you want. You're just lucky to have anything that works, and that's a very healthy thing—especially for people like plastic surgeons, who should be innovators. It's always amazing how in these situations you can get wonderful results with such limited resources, and do

so much in a short time with so many different people—and have a good time yourself. On top of it all, the experience of being there, going someplace and having professional associations with people in that kind of a situation, is a real pleasure.

"Giving Is Living" is part of being an Interplast volunteer. There's no greater joy or greater power, literally, than in giving. That's why we come back; we all want to do that because it's so much fun. Because it brings us great joy.

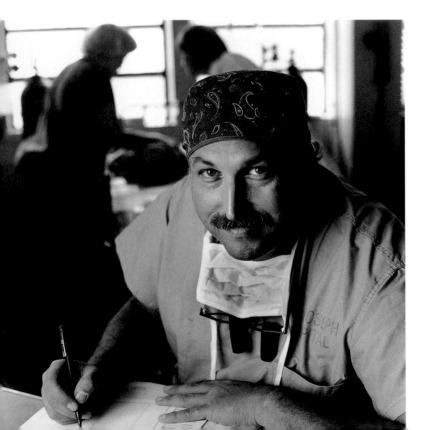

paul

I feel each time I go

PLASTIC SURGEON
KIRKWOOD, MISSOURI

I learn something, sometimes many things. I've tried to learn to do more with less, and not complain about conditions or things I don't have any real control over. I try to emphasize with others that I work with—hospital nurses, OR directors, purchasing people—how we can conserve and do things more efficiently. We're fortunate to have all these supplies; let's not waste them needlessly.

We're so wasteful here in America. Oftentimes, if a procedure's going to take more than an hour or two, they'll send somebody in to give the people who started the case a break. When the case is four, five, six hours long, fine. When the case is only an hour or two long, though, there's no reason to waste another gown, another set of gloves, another everything. A person ought to be able to do a case for an hour or two without a break. I can assure you that rubber gloves and gowns are at a premium in other areas of the world; we shouldn't be tossing them out so someone can have a cigarette only an hour into a case. Yet old habits die hard. It's difficult to change how things have been done for years and years.

On these trips, I've had many patients, or the parents

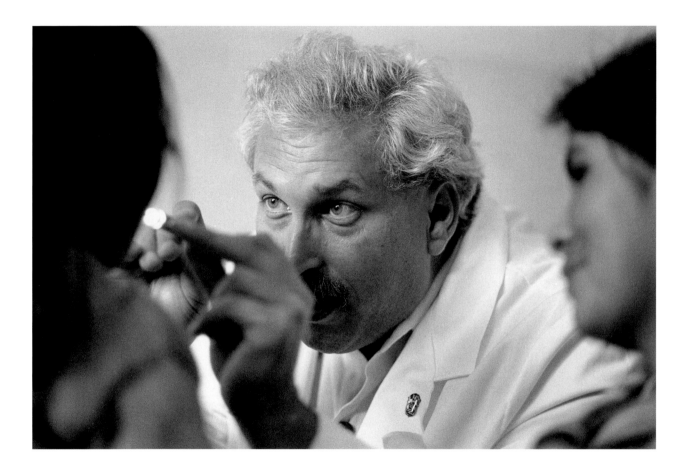

of patients, give me little things—a doll they made, a statue, or a trinket or piece of pottery. Some people don't have the money to go around the block, but they come up with a dollar trinket as a way of saying thanks. On my first trip, I got three or four different little statues, and I had them all lined up on the windowsill in the room where I was staying. One of the anesthesiologists asked me if I was starting my own shrine there.

But, really, just the smile on Mom's face and the look in her eyes—that's all the thanks I go there for. That's what I think really makes the greatest impression on me. I've seen people cry when they first look in a mirror and see their face, their lip repaired. Or see an arm straightened out when it's been at an acute angle for years and years. That's what revitalizes me.

barbara

This was my eighth

RECOVERY ROOM NURSE
SALT LAKE CITY, UTAH

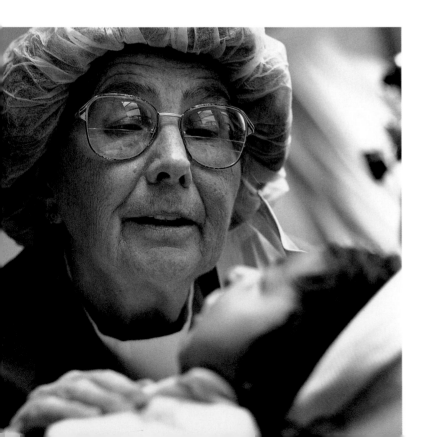

trip, but I've never had such a feeling of . . . just sheer joy, just the joy of being part of that team. And I was a total stranger—I knew no one on the team before I went, before we met in the Dallas airport. But I felt such an integral part of the team right from the start— partly because of the team members themselves; they encompassed me and welcomed me into the group. It was a particularly joyful feeling that maybe a hundred years from now, the world may be different because I had an influence, because something I did was impor- tant in the life of a child. And then to be part of a team that was held in such high esteem by the people there; I've never felt so . . . needed. Does that sound corny?

If there's a common denominator to these trips, it's universal: the love that mothers have for their chil- dren, and the fathers as well. So many times it's the father who's the communicator, because the mother doesn't speak Spanish; particularly in the high moun- tains of Peru, for example, it's the father who speaks the language. They are very concerned about this ter- rible deformity, and they feel guilty, so the thing we try to communicate to them is that it isn't anything *that they've done wrong. But I think the fact that the people are there shows the love that they have for their children.*

Little Stephanie, who had the hand repair, was so darling, and everybody took a shine to her. She was so sweet, and so upbeat, and everybody wanted her to do well. Her mother invited everybody to her home. It wasn't that we didn't want to go, but there was no way we could go. Another one who impressed me was a mother who came, carrying a baby on her back—he was about fifteen months old, and she had a three-month-old baby with a cleft palate—and she was nursing the one baby, and holding another baby on her back; that scene really made an impression on me.

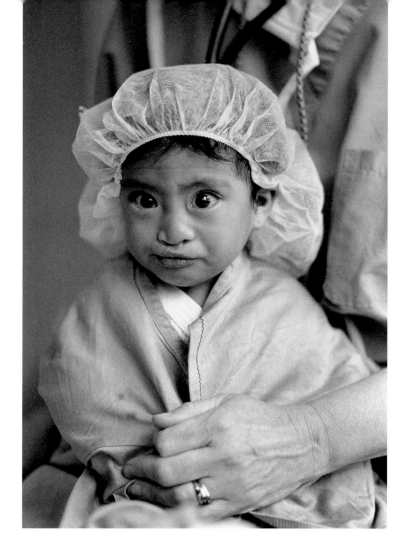

mike

My first trip with

ANESTHESIOLOGIST
PALO ALTO, CALIFORNIA

Interplast, to Ecuador in 1984, was reminiscent almost of boot camp, where you were just so busy every waking moment and sleeping very little—the intensity of the experience was just terrific. When it was over, I remember feeling that anyone who had not been on the trip could not possibly understand all the emotions and feelings that we had. The feeling was that we had worked extremely hard, but had done very good work.

On one of the Vietnam trips, I was making rounds three times a day, so I saw the families and the kids a lot. There was tremendous gratitude from the patients and their families, because I was the doctor who was coming around making their pain go away three times a day and keeping it away. People would routinely give me gifts, or want to take a picture of me with their child.

Their eyes would light up when they saw me. I'd walk into a room at 11:00 at night, it'd be 90 to 93 degrees Fahrenheit in the room, and there would be twenty kids in bed, and another forty people lying on the floor. I'd be stepping over the bodies, but everybody

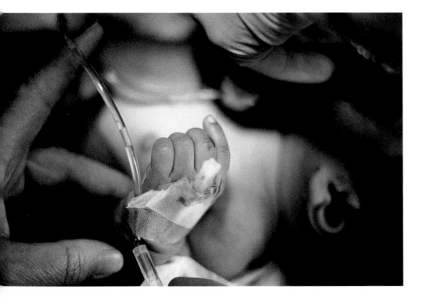

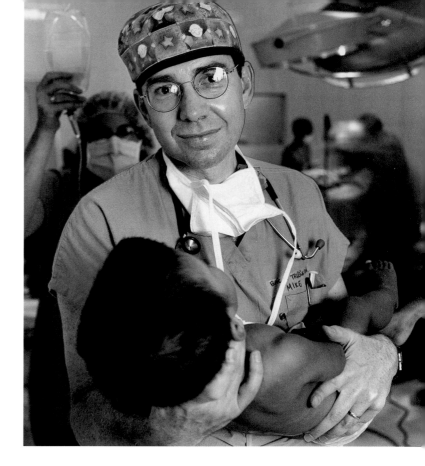

would get up when I came around to their kid. They'd sort of bow, and they were all so grateful. You'd never see something like that in the United States.

I got to know the Vietnamese anesthesia team very well over about a five-year period. I got a tremendous amount of pleasure out of the teaching I did for them, and they really viewed me as an honorary member of their department. That was where I really felt I was giving more. I felt I had a real impact in that teaching situation. I don't like to talk like I'm blowing my own horn, but I think I took them through twenty years of anesthesia techniques in the space of the five years I worked there.

I remember one night my birthday happened to fall while I was there, and I made some mention of it to someone. It was really very sweet because several of the anesthesiologists and nurse anesthetists rode over to our hotel on motorbikes, picked me up, and took me out to celebrate my birthday. It's a moment I've remembered and always will remember. Over the years, I've gotten wedding invitations when some of the nurses have

gotten married, and I've certainly stayed in touch with the anesthesiologists there and consider them to be some of my best friends.

I become very self-conscious when I talk about how we're doing this great work for these people. Clearly I think we are, or I wouldn't be doing it. There are times when you get complications, or it's frustrating. Ultimately, though, I find the work incredibly rewarding.

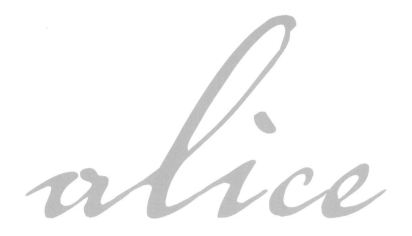

alice

The thing that surprised

me in Vietnam was that there wasn't a lot of resentment in the provinces where we were; we were really welcomed with open arms, and gratefully. I guess I expected to encounter a lot more residual resentment from the war.

PEDIATRICIAN
BERKELEY, CALIFORNIA

I noticed an extraordinary sense of family devotion. I mean, these parents are just tremendously devoted to their kids. I was really struck that, in a country that has so little, they are so rich in love and devotion to their children and their other family members. They sat outside in the rain, waiting for days; they walked hundreds of miles to get there, you know, and that shows a great unity of family and sense of family values.

I remember the grandparents, and aunts and uncles, that whole extended family unit . . . they'd come to the hospital, and sit for hours and days. There was always a family member—or two or three—with each of those kids. It was a phenomenal experience . . . it was like out of some movie.

They were all there, tending their own—no child was left alone. I mean even the little mountain girl—other families kind of adopted her and her mother, even

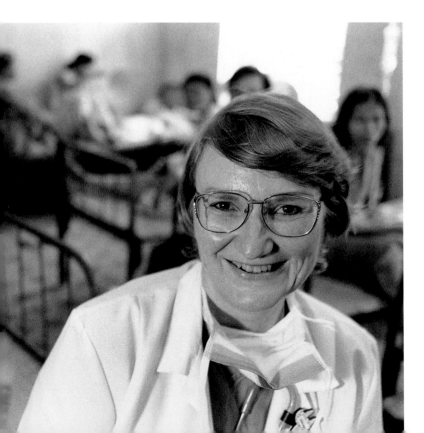

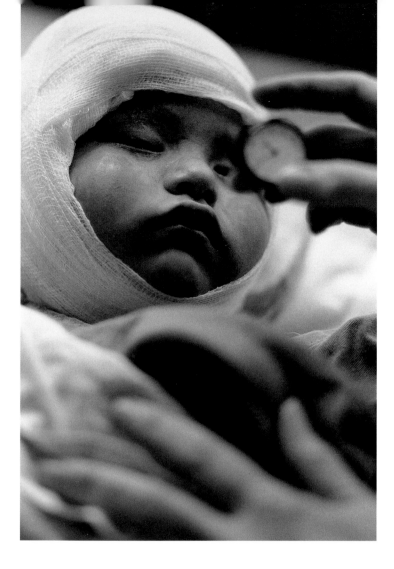

and we have food in the supermarkets—and in the United States you can talk about nutrition to parents and not have them look back blankly at you, saying, "But all I have is rice." We had one baby in Vietnam who was so malnourished that we couldn't do anything. I think this kid was about eighteen months, and was the size of a five- or six-month-old, with a bloated belly, and totally emaciated—clearly starving to death. The mother wanted us to fix what she could see, which was the lip, but she didn't understand that because the child was so malnourished, we couldn't do that. And she was heartbroken. She was trying to breastfeed, but she was malnourished herself. No goats, no cattle. All they ate was vegetables and rice—no protein, no dairy. It was just heartbreaking.

I've found I am now a lot more tolerant of my patients; I don't let little tiny things get to me and ruin my day as much as before. You can't take a lot of things as seriously, because you look back on what this whole country lives with and without every day, and you think, "How can I complain? This could be so much worse."

It really did change me fundamentally from that perspective.

I've tried to communicate this to my patients and parents, to take a little bit of a laid-back attitude when they come in in crisis—or what they think is a crisis, because the kid has had a cold for five days, you know. I have a much calmer approach, and really tend to defuse the situation by saying, "Now wait a minute—think how much worse this could be. You know, this is not the end of the world here. . . ."

though the only one who could speak to her was one guy who was kind of their unofficial translator; they made sure that she got her questions answered, and if she needed anything, they'd come and tug on our sleeve and get someone to come over and take care of her. They really did embrace her, even though she was from the mountains. It was something extraordinary that you just don't see in the United States.

These trips really bring home to me how abundant this country is, and how jaded we are and how much we take for granted. You know, we have clean, dry homes,

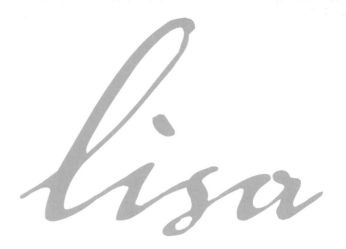

lisa

I find it difficult

OPERATING ROOM NURSE
ST. LOUIS, MISSOURI

to put my feelings into words. Right now I feel there is nothing I might do ever again in my life that can compare to this experience—nothing that will bring me so much. My thoughts are filled with the people I met during the trip; I see their faces all the time; they are in the back of my mind all the time . . . and my memories of them lift my spirits and fill me with a calmness and peace.

I gave so little, but got so much in return—I worked my hours each day, and it felt like such a little part of myself that I was giving, but it meant so much to the people we were helping.

There is so much pain and suffering, but you help one family member, and the love is spread throughout everyone in that family, so you receive love many times over. It truly is multiplied.

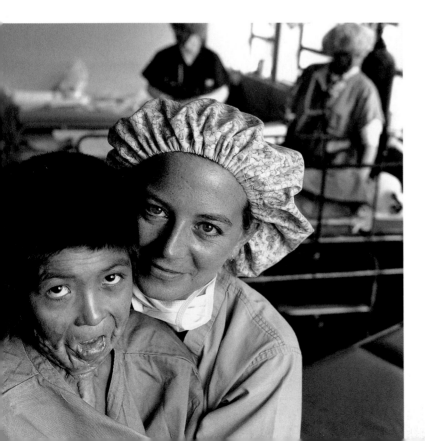

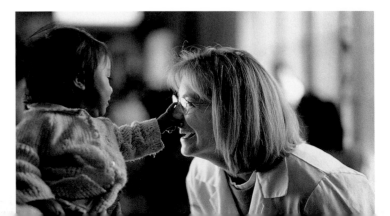

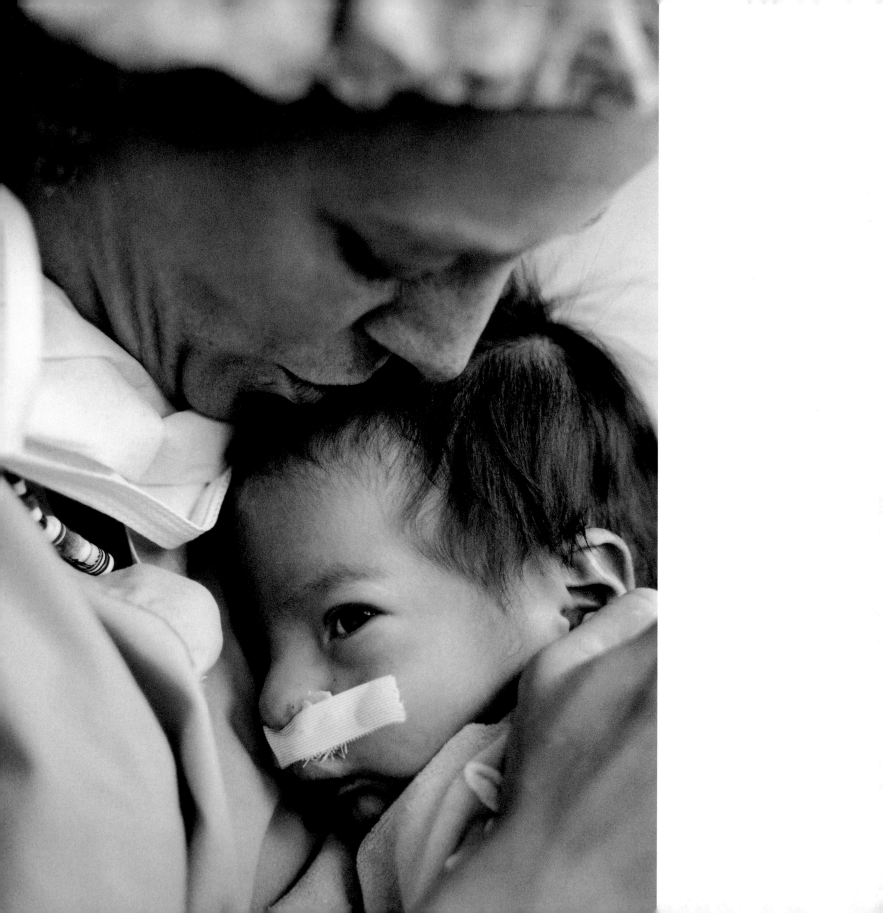

call to action

Greater Than the Individual

Interplast volunteers ask for nothing in return, except the satisfaction that they've done something of value and significance—and yet they gain something. Everyone involved feels the power of giving.

Think of the human body: each cell independently vies for more food and oxygen from the bloodstream, but each also works with others under a central control to maintain a larger organism. A healthy society works similarly, with individuals working for themselves but also providing for something beyond just personal well-being.

When we do something to help others, the recipients obviously benefit. In the long term, though, everyone else gains as well, and the more that is contributed to others' lives, the greater the returning benefits. It's very powerful for the patient, of course, but it's powerful as well for the medical team. It's a complete cycle of giving and receiving, and it grows: besides doing the surgeries themselves, Interplast volunteers also teach other doctors and nurses how to perform the surgeries so that they, in turn, can teach others. Everyone becomes part of the cycle.

Which is what Interplast is about. Helping a child by repairing a cleft lip is a small miracle that happens fifty or a hundred times on every Interplast trip. From a plastic surgeon's standpoint, the procedure is relatively simple—but in that hour or two a patient's life is changed dramatically, for the better and forever.

An equally vital link in that cycle is the financial donor. The first person to donate to Interplast, over thirty years ago, was a philanthropist who gave us $3,000. The money helped us provide thirty-nine surgeries in a little town in Mexico. Interplast volunteers did the surgeries—we were the agents—but the financial support made it all possible.

Since that time, Interplast has performed more than 35,000 surgeries around the world. In a very real sense, that first donor remains part of every one of those small miracles. So does every person who supports Interplast, financially or as a volunteer, or who continues to play a role in sustaining the process. Of course, supporting Interplast is just one way in which people can do something personally important; there are many ways, as individual and distinctive as the people themselves. The crucial thing is to find a way, and to join the endless cycle of giving and receiving.

Donald R. Laub, M.D.
Founder and International Chair, Interplast, Inc.
Los Altos Hills, California
December 1999

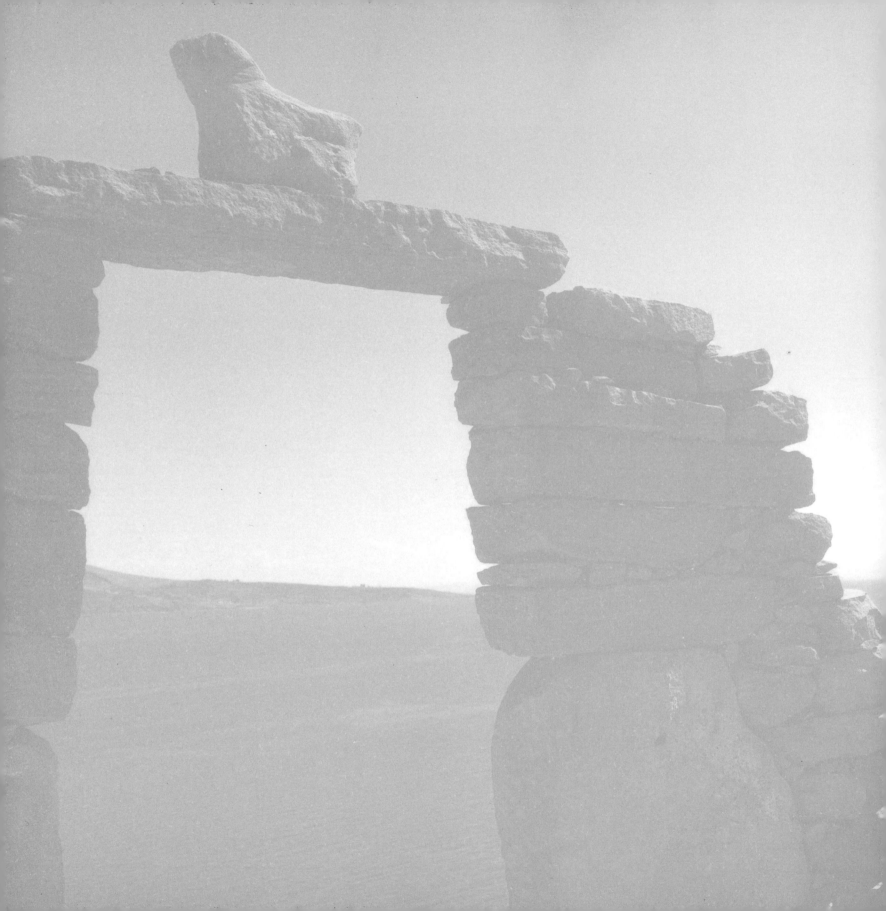